ANNUAL REVIEW OF NURSING RESEARCH

Volume 7, 1989

ANNUAL REVIEW OF
NURSING RESEARCH

Volume 7

Joyce J. Fitzpatrick, Ph.D.
Roma Lee Taunton, Ph.D.
Jeanne Quint Benoliel, D.N.Sc.

Editors

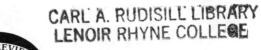
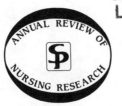

SPRINGER PUBLISHING COMPANY
New York

Order ANNUAL REVIEW OF NURSING RESEARCH, Volume 8, 1990, prior to publication and receive a 10% discount. An order coupon can be found at the back of this volume.

Copyright © 1989 by Springer Publishing Company, Inc.
All rights reserved

Springer Publishing Company, Inc.
536 Broadway
New York, NY 10012

89 90 91 92 93 / 5 4 3 2 1

ISBN-0-8261-4356-3
ISSN-0739-6686

ANNUAL REVIEW OF NURSING RESEARCH is indexed in *Cumulative Index to Nursing and Allied Health Literature* and *Index Medicus.*

Printed in the United States of America

Contents

Preface

Over the years the scientific and professional nursing community has benefitted from the *Annual Review of Nursing Research* series. Through this series authors have contributed to the development of nursing knowledge for the discipline. With the series now well established, there is a firm foundation for the future. We hope that the scientists and professional practitioners in nursing will continue to use these volumes to develop new knowledge, strengthen research, and, ultimately, test the applications in professional practice.

As in previous volumes, research reviewed for Volume 7 follows the established format of five major parts: Nursing Practice, Nursing Care Delivery, Nursing Education, the Profession of Nursing, and Other Research. In each of these areas we identify experts to review the research in a defined topic area.

The chapters under Nursing Practice for the present volume are focused on physiological dimensions. L. Claire Parsons and Pamela Stinson Kidd review neurologic nursing research; Kathleen S. Stone and Barbara Turner review research on endotracheal suctioning; Willa M. Doswell examines physiological stress responses; Joan Shaver and Elizabeth C. Giblin review sleep research; and Elaine L. Larson examines work on infection control. Chapters in this area in Volumes 1 and 4 were focused on human development along the life span, chapters in Volume 2 on the family, chapters in Volume 3 on the community, chapters in Volume 5 on human responses to actual and potential health problems, and chapters in Volume 6 on specific nursing interventions. Authors in Volume 8 also will address physiological aspects of nursing.

In the area of nursing care delivery, Mi Ja Kim analyzes the research on nursing diagnosis, and Susan Boehm examines research on patient contracting. In the section on nursing education, as in previous volumes, there is a focus on areas of specialized clinical education. Cheryl S. Alexander and Karin E. Johnson review research on parent-child nursing education. Research on the profession of nursing includes a chapter by Shaké Ketefian on moral reasoning in nursing and ethical practice.

In the area of other research, one chapter is included in this volume. Carol A. Lindeman reviews research on patient education. In this section we are interested particularly in including international nursing research; we have targeted chapters in future volumes that will be focused on nursing research in other countries.

The success of the *Annual Review* over the past 7 years has been enhanced by the contributions of the distinguished Advisory Board. We express our appreciation to them; their advice and support have been invaluable. We also most gratefully acknowledge the critiques of anonymous reviewers and the editorial and clerical assistance provided by support staff at Case Western Reserve University, the University of Kansas, and the University of Washington.

As always, we welcome readers' comments and suggestions for shaping the upcoming volumes, including identifying potential chapter contributors. Please let us know your interests in contributing to the series and your comments on this volume.

Contributors

Cheryl S. Alexander, Ph.D.
School of Hygiene and Public Health
Johns Hopkins University
Baltimore, Maryland

Susan Boehm, Ph.D.
School of Nursing
University of Michigan
Ann Arbor, Michigan

Willa M. Doswell, Ph.D.
Office of Corporate Nursing Services
New York City Health and Hospitals
    Corporation
New York, New York

Elizabeth C. Giblin, Ed.D.
School of Nursing
University of Washington
Seattle, Washington

Karin E. Johnson
School of Nursing and Health
Sciences
Salisbury State College
Salisbury, Maryland

Shaké Ketefian, Ed.D.
School of Nursing
University of Michigan
Ann Arbor, Michigan

Pamela Stinson Kidd, M.S.N.
College of Nursing
University of Kentucky
Lexington, Kentucky

Mi Ja Kim, Ph.D.
College of Nursing
University of Illinois at Chicago
Chicago, Illinois

Elaine L. Larson, Ph.D.
School of Nursing
Johns Hopkins University
Baltimore, Maryland

Carol A. Lindeman, Ph.D.
School of Nursing
Oregon Health Sciences
    University
Portland, Oregon

L. Claire Parsons, Ph.D.
College of Nursing
University of Arizona
Tucson, Arizona

Joan L. F. Shaver, Ph.D.
School of Nursing
University of Washington
Seattle, Washington

Kathleen S. Stone, Ph.D.
College of Nursing
The Ohio State University
Columbus, Ohio

Barbara Turner, D.N.Sc.
Chief, Clinical Nursing Services
Madigan Army Medical Center
Department of Nursing
Tacoma, Washington

Forthcoming

ANNUAL REVIEW OF
NURSING RESEARCH, Volume 8

Tentative Contents

PART I

Research on Nursing Practice

Chapter 1

Neurologic Nursing Research

L. Claire Parsons
College of Nursing
University of Arizona

Pamela Stinson Kidd
College of Nursing
University of Kentucky-Lexington

CONTENTS

This review covers selected research conducted in neurologic nursing between 1978 and 1987. The majority of the reports reviewed were conducted within the last 5 years. In many cases, the research reports

The authors wish to acknowledge the following people with appreciation and thanks: Terri Britt, R.N., for the collection and initial annotation of materials; Nancy McConaughy for proofreading and editing; and Pat Knight for typing and reproduction.

3

were built on the findings of anecdotal studies originating in the 1960s. Knowledge related to physiologic responses during nursing interventions in persons with intracranial hypertension has evolved from programs of research that began in the 1970s and are still in progress. The studies reviewed were categorized according to the following criteria: patient responses to neurologic injury; factors influencing intracranial pressure; methods and instruments used to assess patient responses; prognostic indicators; and attitudes toward neurologically impaired patients.

Papers chosen for review were selected in a three-step process. Nursing and medical indexes were checked manually for the 1978 to 1987 time period in order to identify potential studies for inclusion. A computer search then was conducted as a way of validating the thoroughness of the manual search. Papers were screened initially to assure that research was reported and then reviewed for the rigor of the research design. The authors have included studies that appeared to represent scholarly endeavors and had clinical implications.

Several consistent factors limited the degree of confidence that can be placed in the findings of the studies reviewed. Many investigators did not address calibration of intracranial pressure monitoring equipment. The samples were small and included a wide variety of craniopathology derived from different mechanisms of injury. Although nursing care activity appeared consistent across samples, medical management differed substantially within and across samples. Variables within studies often were ill defined, and there was a lack of consistency in defining concepts across studies. Lastly, the reliability and validity of questionnaires often were not discussed.

PATIENT RESPONSES TO NEUROLOGIC INJURY

Data exploring patient responses to neurologic injury and to treatment modalities are scarce within nursing. There appears to be a lack of replication of research in this area.

Neurologic trauma in patients continues to be the single most frequently encountered medical problem associated with the nervous system. A prospective study on the neurologically traumatized patient has been described by Rimel (1981). The study was done by dividing patients into severe, moderate, and minor categories with corresponding

Glasgow Coma Scale scores (Teasdale & Jennett, 1974) of 3 to 9, 10 to 12, and 13 to 15 respectively. The purposes of the overall study were to identify the populations with the greatest risk for neurologic trauma, outline treatment strategies, and identify the eventual outcomes of treatment strategies. The data collection tool was used specifically to obtain a descriptive profile of the at-risk patient populations, the mechanisms of injury, the Glasgow Coma Scale scores, the treatment modalities, and the eventual outcomes. By identifying head-injured patients through a daily review of the emergency department admission log and trauma patient charts, 1,330 subjects were classified. Significant descriptive characteristics of the sample included: a greater number of males than females; a higher risk between ages 10 to 30 and over age 65; a higher risk for older adults and single adults; and an annual income of less than $10,000. Thirty-nine percent had been hospitalized previously for a central nervous system injury, and 25% had received professional treatment for alcohol abuse. The most prevalent mechanism of injury was a motor vehicle accident involving a speed greater than 55 mph, injuring a nonrestrained driver in a full-size car. Most injuries occurred on the weekends between 3:00 and 8:00 P.M. Initial Glasgow Coma Scale scores were 8 or less in 25% of the sample, indicating severe neurologic injury. Numerous additional risk factors were identified within the study. The study also provided statistics on various treatment modalities and associated injuries.

Automatic arousal and fear were the focus of a quasi-experimental study conducted by Winters and Padilla (1986) on persons with spinal cord injury. A convenience sample of 45 subjects, 15 with cervical cord injury, 15 with thoracic or lumbar cord injury, and a control group of 15 subjects, viewed a 15-minute horror film. Selection of the control group was not explained in the study. Before subjects viewed the film, pulse rate, blood pressure, and respiratory rate were recorded three times at 5-minute intervals. After hearing an emotionally neutral story, each subject completed a self-rating instrument of fear. Respiratory rate, pulse, and blood pressure were reevaluated during the last 90 seconds of the film, at the completion of the film, and at 5 to 10 minutes postviewing. Subjects completed the self-rating of fear within 10 minutes of viewing the film. A 3 × 4 repeated measures analysis of variance was completed using calculated change scores for time and fear. Results demonstrated significant increases in pulse rate during the film for both the thoracic and lumbar spinal cord injury patients and control subjects. Significant differences in systolic blood pressure, respiratory rate, and self-reports of fear were not present among groups. Subjects with cervical spinal cord injury had the greatest random fluctuations in all parameters. The investigators recommended utilizing other indicators of arousal such as galvanic skin resistance and electromyography in future research. Winters and Padilla (1986) concluded that persons with quadriplegia may have been influenced by fear-based behavior change strategies less than persons with lower spinal cord injury. However, an alternative conclusion could be that persons with cervical spinal cord injury have less control over autonomic function than do persons with thoracic or lumbar cord injuries.

The control of chronic pain has remained a prevalent problem that inflicts high financial cost and suffering. Williams (1984) discussed the use of deep brain stimulation as a modality for managing chronic pain. A case history was presented of a patient with spinal cord injury who had experienced a 20-year history of chronic pain unrelieved by two cordotomies, myelotomy, rhizotomy, and narcotics. Deep brain-stimulating electrodes were implanted in the patient via ventriculography under local anesthesia. Percutaneous leads were connected to the implanted electrodes and affixed to the burr hole using adhesive. The leads connecting the electrodes to the stimulator were brought to the outside of the skin and connected to a temporary transmitter that emitted stimulation pulses from .2 to 1 millisecond duration with a frequency range between 25 and 100 Hertz (cycles per second). After optimum combinations of leads, voltage, and frequency for achieving pain relief were determined, a receiver was implanted subcutaneously in the subclavian region. A receiver cable was tunneled upward and behind the ear through subcutaneous tissue and connected to extensions of the implanted electrodes. The patient could control the system through an external radio-frequency transmitter. The patient obtained pain relief within 15 minutes of activating the transmitter. The pain-free period was maintained for 5 to 6 hours.

The use of deep brain stimulation raises questions for future research. For example, how do particular nursing interventions influence the frequency of required stimulation to obtain pain relief? The impact of other variables such as culture and diagnosis on frequency of deep brain stimulation use also requires investigation.

Snyder (1983a) studied the impact of relaxation on psychosocial functioning in a sample of 32 epileptic patients. An experimental design in which subjects were assigned randomly to a treatment and control group was used. Both groups completed the Washington Psychosocial Seizure Inventory (Dodrill, Batzel, Queissen, & Tomkin, 1980) adapted into a Likert-type format prior to implementation of the treatment. Reliability of the Inventory was evaluated with a correlation coefficient of .84 among raters who evaluated subjects' psychosocial functioning. The raters' scores were correlated with subjects' responses on the Inventory, but validity coefficients were not reported. Members of the experimental group were taught progressive muscle relaxation in six sessions. All subjects kept records of the number of seizures experienced in a 6-month period. Additionally, the experimental group kept a record of the number of times relaxation was used and its effects. Attrition was a problem because only 16 subjects continued in the study for 6 months. Statistical analysis by *t*-test did not reveal significant differences between the experimental and control groups in original scores on the Washington Psychosocial Seizure Inventory, 6-month scores on the instrument, or between the initial and 6-month scores of the experimental group. The investigator made several suggestions for future research. Measurement of another dependent variable such as anxiety might be a more appropriate aim of relaxation than psychosocial functioning. Other methods of teaching relaxation might be more effective than the method used in the study. Converting the Inventory into a Likert-type format may have limited the instrument's capacity for measurement.

FACTORS INFLUENCING INTRACRANIAL PRESSURE

An increasing emphasis in nursing research on factors influencing intracranial pressure has been seen in the last decade. The literature includes studies of environmental, nursing, pharmaceutical, and psychosocial factors. Pediatric as well as adult populations have been the targets of these studies.

Pediatric Populations

The impact of touch on intracranial pressure was investigated by Mitchell, Habermann-Little, Johnson, VanInwegen-Scott, and Tyler (1985), who studied the frequency of spontaneous (procedural and nonprocedural) touch and the effect of investigator touch on intracranial pressure and arterial blood pressure in 13 children aged 7 months to 12 years. These patients had intracranial hypertension secondary to a variety of causes. All children were monitored invasively by epidural fiber optic transducer and intraarterial pressure transducer methods. Terms were defined operationally. Observers sat at each patient's bedside and recorded activity occurrence by use of an investigator-developed tool. Touch was classified into one of four categories: touch alone, touch with talk, touch with procedure, or investigator touch. Interrater reliability was 90% among observers. Standardized investigator touch was accompanied by continuous readings of intracranial pressure and arterial blood pressure for 2 minutes before, 2 minutes during, and 2 minutes after the stroking. Investigators reported that the number of procedural touches did not differ significantly from the number of nonprocedural touches. Intracranial and blood pressure values did not change significantly, beyond an individual's own physical variability, as a result of investigator touch. The investigators concluded that it is safe to increase nonprocedural touching of head-injured children.

Fisher, Frewen, and Swedlow (1982) studied the impact of airway suctioning on nine children, aged 9 months to 12 years, with head trauma; all were intubated and ventilated mechanically. All subjects had intracranial pressure measured invasively with a subarachnoid bolt connected in series to a pressure transducer. End tidal volume of carbon dioxide was measured with an infrared carbon dioxide (CO_2) analyzer. Each subject was studied twice for 30 seconds, once with and once without suctioning. The ordering of the two procedures was done by random assignment. Subjects were hyperventilated 25% longer than normal for 60 seconds prior to and after disconnection from the ventilator. Results demonstrated that mean intracranial pressure increased 5 mm Hg during suctioning and did not change in the nonsuctioning trial. In both trials end tidal volume CO_2 increased during apneic periods, but not significantly. The investigators suggested that increased intracranial pressure during suctioning may have resulted from tracheal stimulation rather than apnea. Because of the small sample size and various treatment modalities in the sample, for example, neuromuscular blockers and osmolar diuretics, this study must be interpreted cautiously.

The impact of head position on intracranial pressure in the neonate was investigated by Goldberg, Joshi, Moscoso, and Castillo (1983). Twenty-six neonates with a mean gestational age of 33 weeks were assigned randomly to one of four independent positions: head turned to the right with bed horizontal (R-0°); head turned to right with head of bed elevated 30 degrees (R-30°); head in midline with bed horizontal (M-0°); and head in midline with head of bed elevated 30 degrees (M-30°). Intracranial pressure was measured with a Ladd monitor fiber optic transducer attached onto skin overlying the anterior fontanelle. Pressure at each position was compared to the mean pressures with head turned to right and bed horizontal. Analysis of variance with multiple range analysis and t-tests were used in data interpretation. The midline-horizontal and midline-elevated positions resulted in lower intracranial pressure values than the right-horizontal and right-elevated positions. If intracranial pressure was greater than or equal to 7 cm H_2O in the right-horizontal or the midline-horizontal positions, elevation of the bed to 30 degrees produced statistically significant decreases in intracranial pressure.

Adult Populations

Findings in several studies have confirmed the deleterious influence of suctioning on intracranial pressure. Nine comatose adult patients with cranial pathology were studied in a descriptive investigation by Snyder (1983b). The influence of nursing activities, environmental factors, and patient states on intracranial pressure was explored. The observer sat with the patient for 4 hours at each data collection period and recorded activities, time, initial intracranial pressure, highest intracranial pressure reached during activity, and length of time the pressure remained elevated. The mean observation period for each subject was 8 to 9 hours. Observers were trained by use of videotape review, and 80% agreement on established criteria was obtained prior to actual data collection. Descriptive statistics were used to analyze the data. The occurrence of patient care activities in rapid succession or simultaneously confounded the results. The data suggested that suctioning, respiratory hygiene, and repositioning increased intracranial pressure the greatest. Because respiratory care was not defined clearly and standardized in the design, additional variables such as flexion of the head may have influenced the results. Although not defined in the design, invasive procedures elevated intracranial pressure for the longest time period. The investigator recommended longitudinal research comparing recovery and prognosis of patients with increased intracranial pressure readings.

In a similar study, Boortz-Marx (1985) investigated the effects of 365 occurrences of health care activities, patient-initiated activities, and environmental stimuli on the intracranial pressure of four subjects with

Glasgow Coma Scale scores of less than 5. Each subject was observed on three occasions for a total of 160 minutes. Subject intracranial pressure was monitored either by subarachnoid bolt or intraventricular catheter. Data were analyzed descriptively. The maximum observed elevation in intracranial pressure occurred with suctioning. Repositioning, physical assessment, and bathing as well as the patient-initiated activities of flexion of extremities, decerebrate movement, flexion or rotation of neck, and spontaneous cough increased intracranial pressure.

Kenning, Toutant, and Saunders (1981) studied the impact of upright patient positioning on intracranial pressure. Twenty-four patients who were monitored invasively for intracranial pressure were placed in a supine position. Recording of intracranial pressure was made for both the supine position and a position with the head and trunk elevated 45 degrees. Standardization of the independent variable was not discussed. Intracranial pressure was reduced in all subjects when the head and trunk were elevated regardless of the initial supine readings.

The effect of kinetic therapy on intracranial pressure was the focus of a study conducted by Gonzalez-Arias, Goldberg, Baumgartner, Hoopes, and Rueben (1983). Ten patients, who were monitored invasively for intracranial pressure, were maintained in constant rotation by placement on a kinetic therapy table. Intracranial pressure was compared in three positions (right to supine, supine to left, and right to left) by using Pearson product moment correlation. Subjects were analyzed, individually and collectively, for differences in intracranial pressure based on position. Table rotation was not associated with differential fluctuations in intracranial pressure.

Bruya (1981) explored the effect of rest periods on intracranial pressure. Twenty adults who experienced head trauma from a variety of etiologies were involved in the study. "Rest" appeared to be defined as absence of nursing care activity. The hypothesis tested in the quasi-experimental design was that the mean pressure and the highest pressure measurement in the treatment subjects who received rest periods would be less than the measurements obtained in the control group. Descriptive statistics were used in the analysis. A comparison of intracranial pressure results in both groups did not support the hypothesis tested; contrary to expectation, intracranial pressure measurements were higher in the subjects who received rest periods. Future researchers could address the meaning of "rest" as defined by the head trauma patient and how long a period of rest is necessary to decrease intracranial pressure.

The effect of presence of the family by the bedside on intracranial pressure was studied by Hendrickson (1987) in a time series quasi-experimental design. Twenty-four subjects over 14 years of age were monitored invasively. Intracranial pressure readings were taken at 15-minute intervals on a 24-hour basis, and 5-minute interval readings were obtained when the family was at the bedside. Data were collected on variables known to influence intracranial pressure, including amount of cerebrospinal fluid drainage, suctioning, nursing procedures, dressing changes, and medications. Data analysis using serial correlation revealed that family presence had a significant positive effect on mean values for intracranial pressure, which decreased from 1.41 mm Hg to 4.24 mm Hg in seven subjects. The study was designed using a nursing approach to a topic that has been studied extensively by use of a medical model.

In a program of research, Mitchell and associates have investigated the effect of nursing activity on intracranial pressure. One of the earliest documented studies on the relationship of nursing activity to intracranial pressure was completed by Mitchell and Mauss (1978). Nine patients who had ventricular catheters in place for pressure-controlled drainage were observed to identify events associated with increases in ventricular fluid pressure that resulted in drainage of ventricular fluid. Activities and level of ventricular fluid were recorded on a checklist, with a 95% interrater agreement obtained. Data were analyzed using the chi-square test with Yates Correction. Rapid eye movement sleep (assessed by observation), suctioning, coughing, painful procedures, and positioning on and off the bedpan were a few of the activities that increased ventricular fluid pressure, as did conducting nursing activities simultaneously. Of interest was the finding that conversation about the patient's condition with the patient or to someone else at the patient's bedside also increased ventricular fluid pressure.

Mitchell, Ozuna, and Lipe (1981) studied the effects on intracranial pressure of moving the patient. A quasi-experimental design was used to determine the variations in ventricular fluid pressure with passive range of motion (hip flexion and extension), head rotation, and turning the body to four positions. Eighteen patients with pressure-controlled external ventriculostomy drainage were studied. Intracranial pressure was measured for 5 minutes preceding and following each nursing activity. Baseline pressure and change in pressure measurements were calculated for each subject and analyzed with descriptive statistics and analysis of variance for repeated measures. In all subjects mean intracranial pressure increased for at least 5 minutes after one of the four turns. Head rotation impacted significantly on intracranial pressure when time was taken into consideration. Accumulative increase in ICP occurred when activities were spaced 15 minutes apart; the increase disappeared with 1-hour spacing. The point in time between 15 and 60 minutes postactivity when intracranial pressure stops increasing was not identified. A limitation of the study was the nonrandomization of sequencing of activities.

The specific impact of head rotation and body positioning on the internal jugular vein was studied by Lipe and Mitchell (1980) in two separate experiments. Internal jugular flow of 10 healthy subjects was monitored by ultrasound for velocity and by echo imaging for cross-sectional lumen size. A random sequence of standardized position changes and head rotations served as the independent variables. The left lateral position had the greatest detrimental effects on cerebral blood flow, manifested by decreased lumen size and increased blood flow velocity. A second experiment with five healthy volunteers was conducted to control more vigorously the degree of head rotation. Degree of head rotation was measured by a goniometer attached to a vertical stand. Results from the second experiment suggested that head rotation of 90 degrees to either side partly or totally occluded the internal jugular vein.

In a series of studies, Parsons investigated the influence of several variables on intracranial pressure. Parsons and Wilson (1984) described the effects of passive position changes on mean intracranial pressure, mean arterial blood pressure, heart rate, and cerebral perfusion pressure in 18 patients with severe head injuries. Six standardized passive position changes were used for all subjects. Subjects had Glasgow Coma Scale scores between 3 and 10 and were monitored invasively for intracranial pressure by an implanted subarachnoid bolt connected to a miniature or standard pressure transducer. Subjects served as their own controls, and data were analyzed by one-way analysis of variance. Results demonstrated that all position changes, except raising the head of the bed, produced increases in mean intracranial pressure, heart rate, and cerebral perfusion pressure. Recovery toward baseline values occurred within 1 minute. The investigators suggested that passive position changes might be performed as long as a patient's baseline intracranial pressure remained less than or equal to 15 mm Hg and cerebral perfusion pressure was maintained greater than 50 mm Hg throughout the position change.

The effect of endotracheal tube suctioning with manual hyperventilation on 20 patients with severe closed head injury was investigated by Parsons and Ouzts-Shogan (1984). Mean intracranial pressure, arterial blood pressure, cerebral perfusion pressure, and heart rate were the dependent variables measured in the same manner as described in Parsons and Wilson (1984). All terms were defined operationally. Subjects were ventilated mechanically with stable hemodynamic (arterial blood pressure ≥ 50 mm Hg) status and had no pulmonary and thoracic complications. Baseline measurements were obtained by nonparticipant observers prior to intervention. The observers recorded the lowest values of the variables obtained during each manual hyperventilation, the highest values obtained during suctioning at four subinterventions, and a final measurement of the variables after the patient had been reconnected to the ventilator for 1 minute. Equipment was calibrated every 4 hours. Data were analyzed between each resting manual hyperventilation and suctioning measurement by independent t-test. Findings suggested that manual hyperventilation after the third endotracheal suctioning should be extended in time in order to decrease arterial blood pressure, intracranial pressure, cerebral perfusion pressure, and heart rate closer to baseline values. The investigators suggested that suctioning could be performed safely upon patients with closed head injury when baseline intracranial pressure was between 0 and 20 mm Hg and cerebral perfusion pressure was 50 mm Hg or greater.

In a quasi-experimental design, Parsons, Peard, and Page (1985) studied the effects of oral hygiene, body hygiene, and indwelling catheter care on the cerebrovascular status of severe closed-head-injured patients. Nineteen patients with Glasgow Coma Scale scores between 3 and 10 constituted the sample. The patients were intubated, ventilated mechanically, and monitored invasively via subarachnoid bolt and intraarterial catheter for intracranial pressure and arterial blood pressure respectively. All equipment was calibrated per protocol; definitions were operationalized, and hygiene interventions standardized. Trained nonparticipant observers obtained baseline measurements of arterial blood pressure, intracranial pressure, cerebral perfusion pressure, and heart rate prior to the initiation of each intervention. During the intervention the highest values for arterial blood pressure, intracranial pressure, and heart rate and the lowest value for cerebral perfusion pressure were obtained. Recovery values were measured at the end of the first minute postcompletion. Interobserver reliability was .80. Analysis of data was performed using analysis of variance. Results revealed that all dependent variables demonstrated significant increases when compared with the respective baseline values for all three interventions. Except for heart rate, recovery values did not differ significantly from baseline values during oral hygiene. Cerebral perfusion pressure was never less than 50 mm Hg with any of the interventions, indicating that these hygiene measures could be performed safely with patients whose resting intracranial pressure was less than 20 mm Hg.

In two recently published reviews of research the influence of nursing care activities on intracranial pressure has been addressed. Both provided excellent summaries of research in this area. Mitchell (1986) discussed nursing research on the impact of patient positioning, turning, head position, suctioning, hygiene measures, and affective sensory stimulation on intracranial pressure. Rudy, Baun, Stone, and Turner (1986) provided a comprehensive review of research mainly on the relationship between endotracheal suctioning and intracranial pressure. In both reviews, as in this analysis, the authors noted that the majority of studies had been focused on describing influences on intracranial pressure. There has been a paucity of researchers investigating the effects of varying nursing intervention strategies intentionally and measuring subsequent modifications in intracranial pressure.

TOOLS USED IN NEUROLOGIC NURSING

Snyder (1986) developed a tool to assess stressors associated with epilepsy. The tool, the Epilepsy Stress Inventory, was a 5-point Likert-type scale used on both outpatient and inpatient epileptic subjects who had a history of seizures for more than 1 year. Stressor was not defined operationally in the study but appeared to reflect patient anxiety related to epilepsy. Six experienced nurses who worked in epilepsy units reviewed the instrument, and all items with 80% or greater agreement were included. A total of 107 subjects completed the Epilepsy Stress Inventory. Test–retest reliability was .55. The stressor with the highest score was "need to take medications regularly," whereas "fear that others will find out about my epilepsy" and "feel rejected by others" were the lowest-ranked stressors. The advantages of the instrument are its ease of administration and speed of completion (5 minutes). The low reliability coefficient may be related to the instability of stressors that epileptic patients experience. Future researchers should concentrate on identifying which stressors can be predicted based on certain disease-related factors.

Two studies have been focused on developing instruments that index factors relating to mental status and physical responses following head injury. Warren and Peck (1984) performed neuropsychological testing on 62 patients who had suffered severe head trauma (Glasgow Coma Scale score of 8 or less) and who were unable to obey simple one-stage commands or utter recognizable words. The aim of the study was to relate neurosurgical and neuropsychological parameters in order to identify the relationship between physical and psychoemotional recovery following head trauma. Patients were compared on common factors that previously had been documented as effects on neurologic outcome. Mean index scores were obtained for each subject on the Glasgow Outcome Scale (Jennett & Bond, 1975) and the Neuropsychological Severity Index. The latter instrument was developed by the investigators and consisted of seven categories: behavior, emotional status, attention/concentration, motor strength, speed and dexterity, verbal and nonverbal memory, and higher level thinking. Reliability and validity data for the Neuropsychological Severity Index were not included. Both tools were administered to the sample 1 year following head injury. Fifty-six percent were rated with the Glasgow Outcome Scale as having had a good recovery, whereas only 8% were rated in this manner by the Neuropsychological Severity Index. The two instruments varied widely in their capacity to describe outcomes.

Interdisciplinary research performed by Turner, Kreutzer, Lent, and Brockett (1984) was performed to develop the Brief Neuropsychological Mental Status Examination. The instrument was intended to identify: (a) early in hospitalization, symptoms that could relate to neuropsychological evaluation three months post-head injury; (b) an early need for speech therapy; and (c) a patient's cognitive status, in order to anticipate patients with a high risk of personal injury and potential learning disabilities. The instrument contains items focused on concentration, sustained attention, orientation, insight, right–left orientation, receptive/expressive language functions, verbal memory, and arithmetic reasoning. The items were derived from subtests of valid tests, that is, the Wechsler Adult Intelligence Scale and Wechsler Memory Scale (Wechsler, 1958) and the Babcock Story Recall (Babcock & Levy, 1940). Eighteen nonrandomized subjects were tested on the Brief Neuropsychological Mental Status Examination, and the instrument was found to be sensitive to cognitive deficits. Impairments most frequently encountered were in immediate and delayed story recall; attention, concentration, and mental tracking; and immediate auditory memory. A contrast group of six patients with brain dysfunction were tested with the instrument. Fifty percent of this sample demonstrated impairment in memory, in sustained attention, and in concentration. The investigators suggested that persons assumed to have minimal potential for injury actually might have limitations not normally assessed. However, caution is necessary in generalizing prematurely on the use of the tool until reliability and validity data are documented. Advantages of the tool are its bedside administration and speed of administration (15 minutes). Further research is necessary to identify the sensitivity of the instrument and the types of patients for whom it might be appropriate.

PROGNOSTIC INDICATORS

Neurologic injuries often are associated with long-term sequelae and an extensive rehabilitation period. Prognostic indicators, which reflect rehabilitation needs and eventual patient outcomes, have not been investigated frequently by nurse researchers.

Head-Injured Patients

The relationship of evoked potentials, the electrical manifestation of the brain's response to an external stimulus, as a noninvasive method of examining functioning of the central nervous system to clinical outcomes in patients with head trauma was investigated by Hummelgard, Martin, and Singer (1984). Two case studies were presented. In the first case study, a 16-year-old boy with an admission Glasgow Coma Scale score of 7 had a brainstem auditory-evoked response that showed a mildly abnormal auditory pathway disturbance. On the sixth day postadmission, evoked responses showed improvement in auditory conduction although the Glasgow Coma Scale score had deteriorated to 4. By the third week postinjury, the patient began to improve and was discharged subsequently to a rehabilitation center. Six months postinjury the patient had made a good recovery as measured by the Glasgow Coma Scale (Jennett & Bond, 1975). In this case, the Glasgow Coma Scale score did not reflect ultimate patient outcome as well as did the evoked potentials.

The second case study involved a 20-year-old male patient with an initial Glasgow Coma Scale score of 5. Brainstem auditory-evoked responses were normal. The right median nerve somatosensory-evoked response demonstrated a moderate left hemispheric disturbance. On the third day postinjury, evoked responses were repeated. A slight improvement in somatosensory pathways was noted; yet the patient's Glasgow Coma Scale score was 7. The patient was transferred 17 days postinjury to a rehabilitation center, and 6 months postinjury had made a good recovery. In this case, the evoked potentials were consistent with the Glasgow Coma Scale score in reflecting prognosis. Further research on the prognostic value of evoked potentials is warranted with larger samples and use of a longitudinal series of evoked responses.

Parsons, Chambers, and Holley-Wilcox (1984) investigated the electrophysiologic changes in the sleep–wake cycle of persons suffering severe head injury. Seventeen subjects with severe head injury were studied in a descriptive correlational design. Electroencephalography, electrooculography, electromyography, electrocardiography, and respiratory rate were used as dependent variables. Twenty-six continuous readings were obtained separately, each over a 24-hour period, and six overnight readings were obtained separately over a 12-hour period. Criteria for interpreting and scoring electroencephalographic readings for these subjects were developed based on the loss and subsequent reappearance of certain electroencephalographic waveforms found in healthy subjects, according to criteria developed by Rechtshaffen and Kales (1968). Numerical values were assigned to the stages of normal sleep and the stages of traumatic coma so that a comparison could be made between an index of staging and the patient's Glasgow Coma Scale score. Correlation between the two measurements was .77. The investigators concluded that lighter sleep stages and wakefulness reappeared in a predictable sequence.

In a retrospective study, Martin (1987) investigated prognostic indicators for 30 children, 15 years of age or younger, who were admitted with a diagnosis of severe head injury. Ten prognostic indicators were correlated with the dependent variables of diffuse cerebral swelling, increased duration of coma, and mortality using nonparametric statistics. Results indicated that age and the absence of corneal reflex were related significantly to occurrence of diffuse brain swelling. Six of the 10 prognostic indicators correlated significantly with duration of coma, whereas 7 out of 10 correlated significantly with mortality. Only absence of corneal reflex correlated significantly with all three dependent variables. Limitations of the study were the small sample size, use of single prognostic indicators, and replication difficulties related to a lack of operationally defined variables. However, the findings provide potential insights for future research on a particular age group that appears to be at high risk for certain outcomes.

Sleep–wake patterns prior to and after cerebral concussion were investigated in a descriptive study (Parsons & Ver Beek, 1982). Seventy-five subjects who had experienced a minor head injury completed an investigator-developed questionnaire 3 months postinjury. The questionnaire contained some items whose stems were modified from the General Sleep Habits Questionnaire developed by Monroe (1967). Pilot data on the psychometric properties of the instrument were not included in the article. Descriptive and inferential statistics were used in the analysis of responses. Several variables were evaluated in regard to their impact on sleep patterns. Patients with more severe injury as measured by Glasgow Coma Scale and length of time in disruption of consciousness showed changes in their sleep–wake patterns. Subjects reported increased arousals, a longer time required to function at peak efficiency upon awakening, increased early morning awakening with failure to return to sleep, and decreased sleep quality. Sleep–wake patterns may serve as an indicator of severity of concussion and subsequent occurrence of postconcussion syndrome. Quantitative electroencephalographic sleep studies are being investigated currently in a similar sample of patients with minor head injuries (Parsons, 1987).

Spinal Injuries

Adelstein and Watson (1983) discussed the impact of using a kinetic treatment table in preventing complications and decreasing length of stay for patients with spinal cord injuries. Four spinal-cord-injured patients were placed on the table, and estimates of time spent in caring for the patients were recorded. These patients were matched for level of injury with spinal-cord-injured patients treated on a regular hospital bed. Definitions of variables were not included in the article. In all but one case, subjects placed on the kinetic treatment table spent less time in acute care than the matched subjects not placed on the table. Statistical analysis was not conducted.

In a preexperimental study of spinal-cord-injured patients, Lyons (1987) investigated factors associated with infection. Data were collected on 77 nonrandomly selected spinal-cord-injured patients and included demographic information, injury level, mobility level, medication, time since injury, and previous infections. Immune response function was measured by several variables including absolute lymphocyte count, gamma globulin, absolute neutrophil count, and albumin. A quasi-control group consisting of 9 bilateral amputees and 10 normal controls was included. Demographic data were obtained by chart review. Statistical analysis was not discussed in detail, but the investigator reported a significant difference in lymphocyte sedimentation rate, alpha-1 globulin, and C-reactive protein between noninfected spinal-cord-injured patients and the controls. An analysis of variance, contrasting the groups with normal and abnormal immune function tests, revealed that administration of diazepam altered lymphocyte counts and acute phase reactants significantly. Multiple regression was used to predict variability in immune function. In spinal-cord-injured patients, infection and characteristics such as level of cord injury and mobility explained the greatest variance. Discriminant function analysis was used to predict infection based on patient characteristics and immune function. C-reactive protein was the most influential variable in predicting infection. Questions generated for future research could be focused on such issues as the influence of diazepam on immune response, further testing of the discriminant function formula to predict patients at high risk for infection, and the time frame in which immune responses become altered.

Ende (1986) replicated a study by Sutcliffe and Vincent (1985) to investigate variables that might be related to length of hospital stay of laminectomy patients. The descriptive study was designed utilizing a retrospective chart review of 65 subjects who had cervical or lumbar laminectomies. Seven variables, employment status, household size, laminectomy level, presence of other medical diagnoses, number of steroid doses, presence of Jackson-Pratt drain, and level of activity, were compared in terms of length of stay by multiple t-test analysis. Hospital stays were longer for patients who were unemployed prior to admission, lived alone, had other medical diagnoses, and had a Jackson-Pratt drain in place during the initial postoperative period. Results support the need for early discharge planning. Future research is needed to assess combinations of these variables in relation to length of stay.

In summary, few studies were found in which prognostic indicators in neurologically injured patients were investigated. Studies on prognostic indicators are a priority need within neurologic nursing research.

ATTITUDES TOWARD NEUROLOGICALLY
IMPAIRED PATIENTS

Mathis (1984) investigated the personal needs of family members of critically ill patients who had sustained an acute brain injury and compared these needs with those of family members of critically ill patients without central nervous system injury. Definitions were operationalized, and sample criteria clarified. A total of 26 subjects were studied; 15 were family members of patients without central nervous system injuries, and 11 were family members of patients with such injuries. Data were collected using a Likert-type scale focused on 45 specific needs. Internal consistency coefficients of .94 and .90, respectively, for family members of critically ill patients with and without central nervous system injury had been established previously using Cronbach's alpha (Cronbach, 1951). Results of a chi-square test on the frequency of identified personal needs within the two groups revealed a statistically significant difference. The 10 most frequently listed needs varied between the two groups, although several similarities were found.

An exploratory study to examine patients who had experienced a cerebrovascular accident (CVA) and had become disabled suddenly was conducted by Davidson and Young (1985). A convenience sample of 29 patients was chosen; of these, 15 had been home from 1 to 7 months, and 14 had been discharged for 12 to 18 months. Subjects were interviewed in their homes using an investigator-developed, open-ended interview guide. Data were analyzed using the grounded theory approach. Descriptive statistics were used to identify frequency of responses and demographic patterns. Based on length of time since discharge, the differences between the two groups were evaluated using the chi-square test. Social patterns changed in that the majority of subjects did not assume any new activities post-CVA; many were unable to resume former activities, and family members were involved in their care. Subjects reported a diminished quality of life. Results of the chi-square analysis demonstrated that recently discharged subjects experienced greater difficulty in getting around the community but had greater functional gains than those who had been home longer.

Noroian and Yasko (1984) studied a convenience sample of 96 nurses to describe the typical neuroscience nurse and the major sources of stress experienced by these nurses. Sample criteria were discussed, and procurement of subjects explained. An investigator-adapted questionnaire, originally designed to survey oncology nurse specialists, was used for data collection. Indexed variables were explained, yet pilot testing of the adapted questionnaire and reliability and validity data were not discussed. Data were analyzed descriptively. The neuroscience nurse profile was a person 34 years old who received an annual salary of $25,635 and who had not been educated in neuroscience nursing as part of a nursing program, but rather after completion of a nursing program. Personal perceptions revealed that the typical neuroscience nurse perceived a moderate to high work stress level, yet was care-oriented and enthusiastic. Most were working in a secondary or tertiary setting. The major sources of identified stress involved problems with administration and policies.

Two studies were designed to investigate nurses' attitudes toward the comatose patient. Loen and Snyder (1980) conducted a pilot study to assess how nurses felt about caring for a long-term comatose patient. Physical care factors that complicated the care of these patients and knowledge deficits in caring for comatose patients also were studied. A nonrandom sample of 91 subjects who had cared for comatose patients completed an investigator-developed questionnaire. Sample criteria were not delineated clearly. Descriptive statistics were used for analysis. Most subjects viewed these patients as challenging and not boring. Thirty-six percent of the subjects advocated rotating the assignment of the comatose patient. Copious tracheal secretions were identified as the greatest problem in physical care. Research concerning different ways of managing physical care factors such as tracheal secretions is needed.

Bell (1986) conducted a similar descriptive study to explore nurses' attitudes in caring for comatose patients. Two additional research questions were focused on (a) the differences in attitudes among nurses working in a surgical intensive care unit, a special care unit, or a general neurosurgical unit, and (b) the differences based on number of comatose patients cared for in the previous year. A nonrandom sample of 48 registered nurses who were working full- or part-time in one of the abovementioned areas and had cared for at least five comatose patients in the previous year participated in the study. The investigator developed an instrument consisting of 25 items written in a semantic differential format. Experts reviewed the instrument for face and content validity. Descriptive statistics and one-way analysis of variance (ANOVA) were used to analyze the data. The subjects viewed the comatose patients as active, animate, progressive, and on the life end of the continuum more than the death end. Yet nurses' attitudes were negative, and discouragement, frustration, and depression were voiced. Most subjects believed that no resuscitative measures should be used in arrest situations with comatose patients. No statistically significant differences in attitudes were present among nurses on the three nursing units. Because 50 ANOVAs were used in the study, the alpha rate or significance level could have escalated, allowing a significant result to occur by chance.

To date, studies have been focused on identifying the personal needs of neurologically impaired patients and their families or the attitudes of nurses when caring for the neurologically impaired patient. Future research in these areas is recommended to describe the impact of various nursing interventions on meeting patient and family needs and subsequently improving satisfaction with nursing care received and patients' quality of life. Whether the attitudes of nurses caring for neurologically impaired patients negatively impact quality of care and whether these attitudes can be changed by identified strategies remains to be investigated.

SUMMARY AND FUTURE RESEARCH DIRECTIONS

A variety of topics in neurologic nursing has been investigated. For this review, studies were classified into the following categories: patient responses to neurologic injury; factors influencing intracranial pressure; instrument development; prognostic indicators; and attitudes toward neurologically impaired patients.

Several areas are suggested for future studies. There is a need to identify individuals with a higher risk than normal of sustaining neurologic injury and patients who have a high risk of death from these injuries. This information could be used to anticipate complications and to develop educational programs aimed at prevention. Research to explore the provision of nursing care to neurologically impaired patients could substantiate staffing requirements empirically and result in a better match between nurse and patient. The effects of nursing behaviors such as therapeutic touch on neurologic status requires investigation. Study of sequencing nursing interventions and the impact of sequencing on intracranial pressure is warranted. Early discharge of the neurologically impaired patient from the hospital may produce problems for the patient and the family. Research in this area might provide nurses with additional information related to rehabilitation.

Last, the identification of outcomes of importance to the patient and the family might assist nurses in planning care during hospitalization. Advancement has been made in neurologic nursing research. There is continuing need to address reliability and validity issues in data collection and to demonstrate greater use of random sampling procedures, clearer definition of variables, and replication of existing studies. To date topics investigated in neurologic nursing reflect a clinical orientation, and many findings are applicable to nursing practice. This result may reflect a sensitivity of researchers to clinicians' needs and priorities.

REFERENCES

Adelstein, W., & Watson, P. (1983). Cervical spine injuries. *Journal of Neurosurgical Nursing, 15,* 65–71.

Babcock, H., & Levy, L. (1940). *The measurement of efficiency of mental functioning (revised examination): Test and manual of directions.* Chicago: C. H. Stoelting

Bell, T. (1986). Nurses' attitudes in caring for the comatose head-injured patient. *Journal of Neuroscience Nursing, 18,* 279–289.

Boortz-Marx, R. (1985). Factors affecting intracranial pressure: A descriptive study. *Journal of Neurosurgical Nursing, 17,* 89–94.

Bruya, M. A. (1981). Planned periods of rest in the intensive care unit: Nursing care activities and intracranial pressure. *Journal of Neurosurgical Nursing, 13,* 184–193.

Cronbach, L. (1951). Coefficient alpha and the internal structure of tests. *Psychometrika, 16,* 297–334.

Davidson, A. W., & Young, C. (1985). Repatterning of stroke rehabilitation clients following return to life in the community. *Journal of Neurosurgical Nursing, 17,* 123–128.

Dodrill, C., Batzel, L., Queissen, H., & Tomkin, N. (1980). An objective method for the assessment of psychological & social problems among epileptics. *Epilepsia, 21,* 123–135.

Ende, R. (1986). The significance of selected variables in laminectomy length of stay. *Journal of Neuroscience Nursing, 18,* 150–152.

Fisher, D. M., Frewen, T., & Swedlow, D. B. (1982). Increase in intracranial pressure during suctioning-stimulation vs. rise in $PaCO_2$. *Anesthesiology, 57,* 416–417.

Goldberg, R., Joshi, A., Moscoso, P., & Castillo, T. (1983). The effect of head position on ICP in the neonate. *Critical Care Medicine, 11,* 428–430.

Gonzalez-Arias, S., Goldberg, M., Baumgartner, R., Hoopes, D., & Rueben, B. (1983). Analysis of the effect of kinetic therapy on ICP in comatose neurosurgical patients. *Neurosurgery, 13,* 654–656.

Hendrickson, S. (1987). Intracranial pressure changes and family presence. *Journal of Neuroscience Nursing, 19,* 14–17.

Hummelgard, A. B., Martin, E. M., & Singer, J. R. (1984). Prognostic value of brainstem auditory evoked potentials in head trauma. *Journal of Neurosurgical Nursing, 16,* 181–187.

Jennett, B., & Bond, M. (1975). Assessment of outcome after severe brain damage. A practical scale. *Lancet, 1,* 480–487.

Kenning, J., Toutant, S., & Saunders, R. (1981). Upright patient positioning in the management of intracranial hypertension. *Surgical Neurology, 15,* 148–152.

Lipe, H., & Mitchell, P. (1980). Positioning the patient with intracranial hypertension: How turning and head rotation affect the internal jugular vein. *Heart & Lung, 9,* 1031–1037.

Loen, M., & Snyder, M. (1980). Care of the long-term comatose patient: A pilot study. *Journal of Neurosurgical Nursing, 12,* 134–137.

Lyons, M. (1987). Immune function in spinal cord injured males. *Journal of Neuroscience Nursing, 19,* 18–23.

Martin, K. M. (1987). Predicting short-term outcome in comatose head-injured children. *Journal of Neuroscience Nursing, 19,* 9–13.

Mathis, M. (1984). Personal needs of family members of critically ill patients with and without acute brain injury. *Journal of Neurosurgical Nursing, 16,* 36–44.

Mitchell, P. H. (1986). Intracranial hypertension: Influence of nursing care activities. *Nursing Clinics of North America, 21,* 563–576.

Mitchell, P. H., Habermann-Little, B., Johnson, F., VanInwegen-Scott, D., & Tyler, D. (1985). Critically ill children: The importance of touch in a high-technology environment. *Nursing Administration Quarterly, 9*(4), 38–46.

Mitchell, P., & Mauss, N. (1978). Relationship of patient–nurse activity to intracranial pressure variations: A pilot study. *Nursing Research, 27,* 4–10.

Mitchell, P., Ozuna, J., & Lipe, H. (1981). Moving the patient in bed: Effects on ICP. *Nursing Research, 30,* 212–218.

Monroe, L. J. (1967). Psychological and physiological differences between good and poor sleepers. *Journal of Abnormal Psychology, 72,* 255–264.

Noroian, E. L., & Yasko, J. M. (1984). A survey of neuroscience nurses. *Journal of Neurosurgical Nursing, 16,* 221–227.

Parsons, L. C. (1987). *Minor head injury: EEG sleep variables and patterns of organization* (Grant No. ROIN32469, University of Arizona). Washington, DC: National Institute of Neurological and Communicative Disorders and Stroke.

Parsons, L. C., Chambers, R., & Holley-Wilcox, P. (1984). Quantitative electrophysiologic changes in the sleep-awake cycle of persons suffering from severe head injury. *Society for Neuroscience Abstracts, 10,* 1000.

Parsons, L. C., & Ouzts-Shogan, J. (1984). The effects of the endotracheal tube suctioning/manual hyperventilation procedure on patients with severe closed head injuries. *Heart & Lung, 13,* 372–380.

Parsons, L. C., Peard, A. L., & Page, M. C. (1985). The effects of hygiene interventions on the cerebrovascular status of severe closed head injured persons. *Research in Nursing and Health, 8,* 173–181.

Parsons, L. C., & Ver Beek, D. (1982). Sleep-awake patterns following cerebral concussion. *Nursing Research, 31,* 260–264.

Parsons, L. C., & Wilson, M. M. (1984). Cerebrovascular status of severe closed head injured patients following passive position changes. *Nursing Research, 33,* 68–75.
Rechtshaffen, A., & Kales, A. (1968). *A manual of standardized terminology, techniques, and scoring system for sleep stages of human subjects* (U.S. Public Health Service Publication No. 204). Washington, DC: U.S. Government Printing Office.
Rimel, R. W. (1981). A prospective study of patients with central nervous system trauma. *Journal of Neurosurgical Nursing, 13,* 132–141.
Rudy, E., Baun, M., Stone, K., & Turner, B. (1986). The relationship between endotracheal suctioning and changes in intracranial pressure: A review of the literature. *Heart & Lung, 15,* 488–494.
Snyder, M. (1983a). Effect of relaxation on psychosocial functioning in persons with epilepsy. *Journal of Neurosurgical Nursing, 15,* 250–254.
Snyder, M. (1983b). Relation of nursing activities to increases in intracranial pressure. *Journal of Advanced Nursing, 8,* 273–279.
Snyder, M. (1986). Stressor inventory for persons with epilepsy. *Journal of Neuroscience Nursing, 18,* 71–73.
Sutcliffe, S. A., & Vincent, P. (1985). Factors related to length of stay of laminectomy patients. *Journal of Neurosurgical Nursing, 17,* 175–178.
Teasdale, G., & Jennett, B. (1974). Assessment of coma and impaired consciousness. A practical scale. *Lancet, 2,* 81–84.
Turner, H. B., Kreutzer, J. S., Lent, B., & Brockett, C. A. (1984). Developing a brief neuropsychological mental status exam: A pilot study. *Journal of Neurosurgical Nursing, 16,* 257–261.
Warren, J. B., & Peck, E. A. (1984). Factors which influence neuropsychological recovery from severe head injury. *Journal of Neurosurgical Nursing, 16,* 248–252.
Wechsler, D. (1958). *The measurement and appraisal of adult intelligence* (4th ed.). Baltimore: Williams & Wilkins.
Williams, A. E. (1984). Deep brain stimulation—a contemporary methodology for chronic pain. *Journal of Neurosurgical Nursing, 16,* 1–9.
Winters, M., & Padilla, G. V. (1986). Autonomic arousal and fear in the spinal cord injured. *Rehabilitation Nursing, 11*(6), 13–17.

Chapter 2

Endotracheal Suctioning

KATHLEEN S. STONE
COLLEGE OF NURSING
OHIO STATE UNIVERSITY

BARBARA TURNER
CHIEF, CLINICAL NURSING SERVICES
MADIGAN ARMY MEDICAL CENTER
DEPARTMENT OF NURSING

CONTENTS

Endotracheal suctioning (ETS) is a procedure performed by nurses to remove secretions and debris from the tracheobronchial tree through mechanical aspiration. Endotracheal intubation prohibits an effective cough because of an open glottis and prevents the mucociliary clearing mechanism, resulting in secretions "pooling" at or near the tip of the endotracheal tube. The endotracheal tube itself may act as an irritant, thus increasing secretions. As these secretions accumulate, they may

27

block or partially occlude the endotracheal tube. Removal of tracheo-bronchial secretions promotes airway patency, thus facilitating oxygenation and ventilation. Intubated patients may be subjected to endotracheal suctioning (ETS) as frequently as every 15 min but more usually every 1 or 2 hours or as needed to maintain airway patency and promote optimal ventilation. The basic endotracheal suctioning procedure consists of inserting a suction catheter into the trachea followed by the application of negative pressure as the catheter is withdrawn. There are, however, many variations on the basic procedure. These include saline instillation for the purpose of irrigation, hyperoxygenation (increased inspired oxygen), hyperventilation (increased respiratory rate), hyperinflation (volume of inspired air greater than baseline tidal volume), and use of a modified endotracheal tube adapter to permit suctioning while on the ventilator. Additional variations associated with the suction catheter include: the application of negative pressure intermittently versus continuously, rotation of the suction catheter upon removal, and head rotation to assist bronchus entry.

Over the past 40 years endotracheal suctioning techniques have been studied descriptively and experimentally by a number of health care professionals including physicians, nurses, and, most recently, respiratory therapists. Nonnursing literature was included in this review, as the early research laid the groundwork for nursing studies. Through a MEDLINE search of variables associated with the endotracheal suctioning procedure and current investigators' names from 1930 through 1987, 163 published research articles were identified. The main topical areas of research include: (a) complications, (b) techniques to alleviate hypoxia, (c) negative airway pressure, (d) intermittent versus continuous negative pressure application, (e) bronchus entry, (f) tracheal tissue damage, (g) secretion recovery, (h) predictors of the need for endotracheal suctioning, and (i) suctioning protocols. The focus of this review is limited to the documented complications associated with ETS and the techniques that have been investigated to relieve the most common complication, hypoxemia, in adults and newborns.

SIMILARITIES AND DIFFERENCES IN ADULT AND NEONATE

When reviewing the complications and current techniques to relieve ETS-induced hypoxemia, similarities and differences between an adult and a newborn are important considerations. The most common reasons for endotracheal intubation in both adults and newborns are acute and chronic respiratory failure; however, the causes of the respiratory failure differ greatly. In its most dramatic form, acute adult respiratory failure is typified by Adult Respiratory Distress Syndrome (ARDS). The initiating mechanisms of the syndrome are quite heterogeneous and range from severe or prolonged hypotension to inhaled irritants in adults. A wide variety of chronic disorders with acute exacerbations can develop into acute respiratory insufficiency. These include chronic bronchitis, emphysema, cor pulmonale with pulmonary edema, status asthmaticus, pneumonia, and neurological deficits such as myasthenia gravis or Guillain-Barré Syndrome.

In newborns, a large number of congenital or acquired abnormalities cause respiratory failure, the most common being respiratory distress syndrome (RDS) or hyaline membrane disease. A syndrome of chronic lung disease in the newborn, bronchopulmonary dysplasia, occurs in survivors of RDS who have been ventilated with enriched oxygen mixtures.

Hyperoxygenation (increasing the concentration of inspired oxygen), a technique to relieve ETS-induced hypoxemia, has been examined experimentally at 20% above baseline and most often at 100% in adults. Oxygen toxicity resulting in retinopathy of prematurity (retrolental fibroplasia) (Phelps, 1987) and bronchopulmonary dysplasia (Fox, Morray, & Martin, 1987) are well documented in the newborn. As a result, hyperoxygenation to relieve ETS-induced hypoxemia in the newborn has been tested at 10% to 20% above baseline, which is considerably less than with an adult. The technique for monitoring the efficacy of hyperoxygenation in preventing ETS-induced hypoxemia is measurement of arterial blood gases in the adult and noninvasive oximetry, which measures oxygen saturation (SaO_2). Because of the small blood volume in the newborn, continuous noninvasive oxygen monitoring using the transcutaneous oxygen electrode (to measure transcutaneous oxygen tension, $tcPO_2$) or oximetry (to measure SaO_2) is the preferred technique. Continuous monitoring of oxygenation throughout the entire suctioning episode has an advantage over periodic arterial blood gases. However, the reliability and validity of noninvasive techniques are dependent upon adequate peripheral skin perfusion, which is frequently compromised in critically ill adults and newborns.

Another dramatic difference between the two populations is physical size. The typical 70 kg man has an average total lung capacity of 6 L, whereas the typical 1000-g premature infant has a lung capacity of 60 cc. Hyperinflation, the volume of inspired air greater than baseline tidal volume, has been investigated extensively and found to be effective in preventing suction-induced hypoxemia in an adult (Baun & Flones, 1984; Boutros, 1970; Fell & Cheney, 1971; Kergin, Bean, & Paul, 1948; Langrehr, Washburn & Guthrie, 1981; Naigow & Powaser, 1977; Skelley, Deeren, & Powaser, 1980). Hyperinflation in the newborn causes overextension of normal alveoli and expansion of atelectic alveoli, which may result in the disruption of the alveolar wall resulting in air leaks or a pneumothorax. For this reason, hyperventilation or increased respiratory rate has been examined extensively in newborns (Cunningham, Baun, & Nelson, 1983; Norris, Campbell & Brenkert, 1982; Raval, Mora, Yeh, & Pildes, 1980; Simbruner et al., 1981). For the adult, endotracheal tubes commonly range from 7 to 9 mm and the suction catheters from 10 to 14 French (Fr.). For newborns, the endotracheal tubes are small, ranging from 2.5 mm to 4.0 mm, thus limiting the size of the suction catheter than can be inserted to sizes 5 Fr. through 8 Fr. In adult patients it is recommended that the suction catheter occlude no more than one half of the diameter of the endotracheal tube to permit the inflow of environmental oxygen while alveolar gas is being removed simultaneously during suctioning (Rosen & Hillard, 1962).

Because of the restricted size of the endotracheal tube, this ratio is not practical in the newborn. Use of the largest catheter that can fit through the endotracheal tube limits the flow of air around the tube but increases the amount of secretions that can be removed. A small suction catheter-to-endotracheal tube ratio would allow airflow around the tube but would decrease the amount of secretions removed by an exponential factor of four to five (Walters & Hartwig, 1979). One then is faced with choosing between restricted removal of secretions or restricted airflow.

Because of the distinct differences between the adult and the newborn relative to pathological process and physical size, experimentally tested endotracheal suction techniques should be developed taking these differences into account. A review of ETS complications and the techniques to alleviate hypoxemia provided evidence that many of the techniques that have been investigated in the adult have been applied directly to the newborn without considering these differences.

COMPLICATIONS ASSOCIATED WITH ENDOTRACHEAL SUCTIONING

In adults, endotracheal suctioning is not a benign procedure. It has been associated with harmful sequelae including hypoxemia (Berman & Stahl, 1968; Boutros, 1970; Urban & Weitzner, 1969), atelectasis (Brandstater & Muallem, 1969; Rosen & Hillard, 1962), bronchoconstriction (Widdicombe, 1954), hypotension (Goodnough, 1985), increased intracranial pressure (Parsons & Shogan, 1984), cardiac arrhythmias (Shim, Fine, Fernandez, & Williams, 1969), and, in some cases, cardiac arrest and death (Marx et al., 1968). Sequelae may be related to the decrease in arterial oxygen levels associated with aspiration of alveolar gas (Kergin et al., 1948), disruption of mechanical ventilation (Ehrhart, Hofman, & Loveland, 1981), and increased intrathoracic pressure (Criley, Blaufuss, & Kissel, 1976; Rudikoff, Maughan, Effron, Freund, & Weisfeldt, 1980).

In the newborn, complications associated with endotracheal suctioning include mucosal necrosis (Fiske & Baker, 1975; Stavis & Krauss, 1980), tracheal lesions (Stavis & Krauss, 1980), bacteremia (Storm, 1980), esophageal perforations (Stavis & Krauss, 1980), pneumothorax (Stavis & Krauss, 1980), atelectasis (Brandstater & Muallem, 1969), increased intracranial pressure (Fanconi & Duc, 1987; Perlman & Volpe, 1983), introduction of a foreign body (Schreiner, Smith, & Gresham, 1976), cardiac arrhythmias (Cabal et al., 1979), and hypoxemia (Cunningham et al., 1983).

TECHNIQUES TO MINIMIZE COMPLICATIONS

The major endotracheal suctioning variables under investigation in both adults and newborns are hyperoxygenation (increased inspired oxygen), hyperventilation (increased respiratory rate), hyperinflation (volume of inspired air greater than baseline tidal volume), and the use of adapters for endotracheal suctioning to maintain continuous ventilation during the procedure. In many of the studies a combination of techniques such as hyperoxygenation/hyperventilation or hyperoxygenation/hyperinflation has been examined. For the review, the studies have been classified systematically based on the major technique examined.

Hyperoxygenation

One of the earliest techniques used in both adults and neonates to relieve the hypoxia associated with ETS was hyperoxygenation. Hyperoxygenation is defined as an increase in the concentration of inspired oxygen (FIO_2) that can be administered prior to (preoxygenation), during (insufflation), and after (postoxygenation) suctioning. Supplemental oxygen can be administered through the ventilator or suctioning catheter (insufflation) or by removing the patient from the ventilator and using a manual resuscitation bag (MRB).

Delivery of supplemental oxygen using the ventilator or MRB has advantages and disadvantages. Ventilator administration has the advantage of being able to preset the rate, volume, and pattern of the hyperoxygenation breath using the manual "sigh" on the ventilator. However, increasing the oxygen concentration on the ventilator requires a "bleed time" or "washout time" for the increased oxygen concentration to rise in the ventilator tubing and to reach the subject. This "washout time" is variable and dependent upon the rate, flow, and tidal volume settings on the ventilator as well as the length and diameter of the ventilator tubing. Hyperoxygenation on the ventilator is advantageous in that positive end-expiratory pressure (PEEP) used in adults and newborns and positive inspiratory pressure (PIP) in the newborn can be maintained. Hyperoxygenation using the MRB requires that the subject be removed from the ventilator and placed on the MRB, thereby losing PEEP and PIP. A consistent elevated oxygen concentration using the MRB is dependent upon the oxygen flow rate, size of the reservoir, and the rate of compression to allow adequate refill of the bag (Preusser, 1985). A severe limitation of the MRB is the variability in the volumes and pressures generated by the operator when delivering the hyperoxygenation breaths. In evaluating the research on the efficacy of hyperoxygenation using the ventilator or the MRB to relieve ETS-induced hypoxemia, the inherent variability of the delivery systems must be considered.

Adlkofer and Powaser (1978) examined the effects of current ETS techniques on arterial oxygen levels (PaO_2) in 64 critically ill but stable patients. Fifty-four of the patients were suctioned without receiving some form of preoxygenation. Ten patients were preoxygenated either by means of the "sigh" control on the mechanical ventilator without increasing the FIO_2 or by use of the MRB connected to an oxygen source with an unspecified concentration of oxygen. The patients who were not preoxygenated had a significant fall in PaO_2 during the first suction pass ($p < .001$) with a mean decrease of 11.6

mm Hg at 60 sec postsuctioning. In contrast, the patients who were preoxygenated by some technique that was not specified did not have a statistically significant change in PaO_2 after the first or second suction pass, with a mean decrease in PaO_2 of 3.1 mm Hg at 60 sec (Riegel & Forshee, 1985).

Simultaneous insufflation of oxygen into the trachea through a double-lumen catheter while suctioning is another technique to reduce ETS-induced hypoxemia. Investigators using oxygen insufflation techniques have reported conflicting results. Berman and Stahl (1968) compared PaO_2 levels following ETS using a conventional catheter in patients inspiring room air alone to insufflation at an oxygen flow rate of 5 L/min in 12 postoperative subjects. ETS with room air resulted in PaO_2 values 1 to 23 mm Hg below resting values, while insufflation raised oxygen levels 68 mm Hg. However, in these experiments the application of negative pressure varied from 15 to 45 sec. Boba, Cincotti, Piazza, and Landmesser (1959) reported an average 16% drop in oxygen saturation with ETS compared to an average 5% drop in oxygen saturation with oxygen insufflation (4 L/min) and ETS in 15 healthy male subjects undergoing minor surgery. Fell and Cheney (1971) examined the effectiveness of oxygen insufflation at 5 L/min in five healthy, anesthetized, spontaneously breathing dogs and in 18 patients with varying degrees of respiratory failure. Results of the animal study confirmed that insufflation was effective in preventing the fall in PaO_2 with ETS, whereas insufflation was not effective in retarding the fall in PaO_2 during ETS in human adults with respiratory failure. The investigators suggested that the conflicting results might be caused by atelectasis with shunt in the human subjects. Langrehr et al. (1981) found oxygen insufflation at 10 to 15 L/min prevented a significant change in mean PaO_2 from control levels at all sampling times in 10 postcardiac surgery patients with relatively healthy lungs.

Until recently, insufflation as a technique to reduce ETS-induced hypoxemia has been examined only in the research laboratory and has not been used clinically because of problems in manufacturing a 14 Fr. double-lumen extruded catheter. Bodai, Walton, Briggs and Goldstein (1987) reported results of a study using the new Jinotti Twin Care Suction Catheter, which permits oxygen insufflation at 15 L/min during insertion and withdrawal of the catheter but not during the application of negative pressure. They evaluated 24 patients with "diverse" disease processes. The subjects were assigned randomly to three groups. The treatment for Group I was preoxygenation/hyperinflation and suction with and without oxygen insufflation. Three lung hyperinflation breaths were administered using an MRB at 1.0 to 1.15 L with 100% oxygen followed by 15 sec of suction and repeated three times. Group I subjects were classified by the investigators as having moderate respiratory failure based on an average baseline FIO_2 of 0.43 and four of the six subjects on PEEP. In this group both preoxygenation/hyperinflation with and without insufflation increased PaO_2 levels. The treatment for Group II was a comparison of preoxygenation/hyperinflation and suction to oxygen insufflation/suction alone. The subjects were classified by the investigators as having moderate respiratory failure as evidenced by an average baseline FIO_2 of 0.47, and 9 of the 12 subjects required PEEP. In Group II, both techniques (preoxygenation/hyperinflation and insufflation) resulted in an average decline of -10 ± 25 mm Hg PaO_2 immediately after suctioning. The treatment for Group III was a comparison of suctioning with and without oxygen insufflation using an adapter to maintain connection to the ventilator. Group III had more severe respiratory failure evidenced by an average baseline FIO_2 of 0.48, and all subjects were on PEEP. In Group III, ETS on the ventilator using the adapter and oxygen insufflation using the adapter maintained PaO_2 values above control values at all times. The investigators concluded that the results in Groups I and II showed that insufflation alone could be as effective as preoxygenation and hyperinflation; however, some patients (Group II) were more sensitive and their responses appeared to be more patient-specific than protocol-specific and called into question the averaging of patient data. Therefore, whereas Group II showed comparability of insufflation to preoxygenation/hyperinflation, Bodai et al. (1987) could not conclude persuasively that either protocol is safe for all patients.

The difficulty in drawing conclusions regarding the effectiveness of oxygen insufflation to prevent suction-induced hypoxemia relates to the variability in the amount of oxygen insufflated 4 to 15 L/min and the diversity of subjects tested. The latter ranged from healthy anesthetized subjects to subjects with severe respiratory failure.

Hyperoxygenation/Hyperventilation

Downes, Wilson, and Goodson (1961) examined the effect of 15 sec of hyperventilation with oxygen in preventing arterial oxygen desaturation during apnea and apnea with ETS in 11 anesthetized adult patients undergoing pulmonary resection with the pleura closed or open. One minute of apnea resulted in a mean decrease of 8% oxygen saturation (SaO_2), whereas hyperventilation with oxygen 15 sec prior to 1 min of apnea resulted in a 2% rise in SaO_2 when the pleura was closed. ETS during apnea did not alter the changes in SaO_2 significantly ($p < .5$). Several methodological issues in this study should be noted. The oxygen concentration of the inspired air (FIO_2) was not stated; the instrumentation to measure SaO_2 has been perfected, and there were only 4 min between experimental trials, which is insufficient to permit equilibration of arterial oxygen levels to baseline levels.

While hyperoxygenation/hyperventilation rarely is used in adults, it is used commonly in neonates for reasons previously discussed. Raval et al. (1980) investigated the effects of endotracheal suctioning, chest physiotherapy, and oral suctioning on transcutaneous oxygen tension ($tcPO_2$) in six preterm and one term infants who were ventilated manually. The endotracheal suctioning procedure consisted of hyperoxygenation and hyperventilation combined into three different suctioning procedures. The first procedure consisted of instilling 0.9 ml of NaCl into the endotracheal tube, followed by hand ventilation for 3 breaths, suctioning for 10 sec, which was repeated three times for each suctioning episode. The second procedure consisted of increasing the oxygen by 10% and hand ventilating for 60 sec prior to carrying out the first procedure. The number of breaths given in the 60-sec period was not reported. The third variation was identical to the second with the exception that the oxygen was increased to 100%. Oxygenation was measured transcutaneously by a heated electrode placed on the infant.

The investigators noted that the first suctioning procedure significantly decreased the $tcPO_2$ for 35 to 425 sec; in contrast, there were no significant changes in $tcPO_2$ levels with the second procedure until the third repetition. At this time $tcPO_2$ levels increased above baseline. The third procedure produced hyperoxic $tcPO_2$ levels. Raval and associates (1980) recommended that increased oxygen of 10% and hyperventilation be used when the baseline PaO_2 is unknown or normal and that 100% oxygen be used when the baseline PaO_2 is hypoxemic.

Simbruner et al. (1981) examined the effects of tracheal suction using an MRB with 100% oxygen on $tcPO_2$, heart rate, and blood pressure in two groups of five intubated infants; infants in one group weighed less than 1250 g, and in the other they weighed over 1750 g. There was no effort made to control the suctioning procedure by the nurses and, as the investigators noted, some of the nurses were experienced whereas others were not. The procedure was performed using 0.5 ml of normal saline followed by hand ventilation with 100%

oxygen, then suctioning using 200 cm H_2O. There was a decrease in $tcPO_2$ and heart rate with an increase in blood pressure during suctioning, but these trends were reversed with bag ventilation. Five min after bag ventilation the $tcPO_2$ and blood pressure were higher than during the control period. There was no correlation between the duration of disconnection from the ventilator and the extent of $tcPO_2$ fall. The length of time that suction was applied was not reported. The investigators noted that severity of disease was the main determinant of the fall in $tcPO_2$ rather than the weight of the infant. Those infants with higher FIO_2 and controlled ventilation were affected to a greater extent than those on intermittent mandatory ventilation.

Using a quasi-experimental design, the three nursing procedures of endotracheal suctioning, heelstick, and repositioning were examined for the effects on $tcPO_2$ in 25 intubated and ventilated premature infants (Norris et al., 1982). Suctioning produced the largest fall in $tcPO_2$ and resulted in the second-longest recovery time of the three procedures. The suctioning procedure was not described in sufficient detail to permit replication or evaluation of the procedure. It was not clear whether the three procedures were administered randomly to allow for exclusion of systematic bias. One confounding factor that can be determined from the report is that the endotracheal suctioning procedure involved movement of the head and thorax, thus including components of the repositioning variable. The effect of the repositioning component on ETS was not addressed.

In a study of eight premature infants, three with respiratory distress syndrome and five with other pulmonary disorders, two concentrations of supplemental oxygen and two inflation times were studied for the effects on heart rate and $tcPO_2$ (Cunningham et al., 1983). The suctioning procedure consisted of a period of ventilation with an MRB followed by 15 sec of nonventilation and 3 sec of 80 to 100 cm of H_2O-applied negative pressure. Four variations were used with the MRB: (a) 10% greater supplemental oxygen given with 5 breaths in 15 sec, (b) 20% greater supplemental oxygen given with 5 breaths in 15 sec, (c) 10% greater supplemental oxygen given with 10 breaths in 30 sec, and (d) 20% greater supplemental oxygen given with 10 breaths in 30 sec.

Infants with RDS responded to ETS with steady decreases in $tcPO_2$ that were not reversed by ventilation. The infants without RDS had $tcPO_2$ levels that fluctuated around the baseline or became elevated above baseline. The authors recommended that 20% supplemental oxygen be given with 5 breaths in 15 sec for infants ventilated for reasons other than RDS. None of the FIO_2/inflation combinations prevented the drop in $tcPO_2$ for infants with RDS.

Hyperoxygenation/Hyperinflation

Kergin et al. (1948) discovered that suctioning patients caused oxygen saturation to decrease 25 to 30%, followed by a slow rise back to baseline over a 3-min period. This reoxygenation period was shortened to 10 sec when a positive pressure of 15 mm Hg was applied to the lungs via an MRB. Boutros (1970) examined arterial oxygenation during endotracheal suctioning and for 3 min after in 22 anesthetized and paralyzed patients with no known pulmonary disease. He demonstrated that one hyperinflation sustained for 10 sec after suctioning resulted in a significantly smaller decrease in PaO_2. The volume of the hyperinflation breath was not stated in the study report, nor was the concentration of oxygen in the inspired air. Vigorous hyperinflation for one min at 100% oxygen was examined by Fell and Cheney (1971) and found to be successful in elevating PaO_2 levels when followed by 15 sec of endotracheal suctioning in 20 subjects with varying degrees of respiratory failure. There were several methodological problems in this study: (a) 10 of the 20 subjects were already being maintained on 100% oxygen before the hyperinflation with 100% oxygen; (b) the volume of the "vigorous" hyperinflation breaths was not stated in this report; and (c) the $PaCO_2$ and pH values were not reported, so a full evaluation of the effect of "vigorous" hyperinflation could not be determined.

Naigow and Powaser (1977) examined the effects of five different suction procedures in two spontaneously breathing anesthetized dogs studied at weekly intervals for 5 weeks. Five randomly ordered suction variations were tested: (a) suction alone; (b) 100% oxygen given by means of a nonrebreathing reservoir bag connected to the endotracheal tube for 3 min; (c) hyperinflation (tidal volume 300 to 400cc) with room air for 5 min postsuctioning; (d) 100% oxygen by hyperinflation for 3 min prior to suctioning; and (e) 100% oxygen by hyperinflation before, during, and after suctioning. ETS alone for 15 sec produced a significant decrease in PaO_2 ($p < .001$). Oxygen at 100% given 3 min prior to suctioning raised oxygen levels ($p < .001$) but did not prevent the fall in oxygen below control postsuctioning. Hyperinflation with room air for 5 min after suction raised PaO_2 levels above control after suction but not during suction.

Administering 100% oxygen prior to suction raised PaO_2 levels after suction, but PaO_2 levels fell below control at 5 min. Hyperinflation at 100% oxygen before, during, and after suction caused PaO_2 levels to remain elevated at all times. This study was performed in dogs with healthy lungs; further testing of these protocols in clinical subjects with varying pulmonary dysfunction is required before recommendations can be made.

In 5 trials, Skelley, Deeren, and Powaser (1980) compared one versus three hyperinflation (1.5 tidal volume) breaths at 100% oxygen prior to suctioning in 3 dogs and 11 postcardiac surgery patients. No preoxygenation resulted in a fall in PaO_2 immediately after suctioning in both dogs and humans. Both one and three hyperinflation breaths prior to suctioning raised the PaO_2 levels in dogs and humans, with the three hyperinflations producing the greatest increase. The increase in PaO_2 in the human subjects was less than in the dogs, and the investigators speculated that it might be because of a greater pulmonary shunt.

Langrehr et al. (1981) examined the effect of one versus three lung hyperinflation breaths at 1.5 tidal volume with 100% oxygen prior to ETS in 10 postcardiac surgery patients. One hyperinflation prior to suctioning produced a significant rise ($p < .05$) in PaO_2, which fell below control levels by 30 sec and remained below control at 300 sec. Three hyperinflations resulted in a rise in PaO_2 immediately following suctioning ($p < .01$), followed by a fall below control at 30 sec and a return to control levels by 300 sec. The investigators hypothesized that the rapid fall in PaO_2 at 30 sec might be because of an adverse hemodynamic effect of lung hyperinflation resulting in decreased blood return to the right atrium or negative airway pressure.

Baun and Flones (1984) examined the effects of three sequential suctioning episodes in six anesthetized dogs. Three suction protocols were tested in a Latin Square design. In protocol A the animals received 15 sec of room air through the ventilator prior to and following three sequential suction passes, which resulted in a maximum mean decrease of 20 mm Hg PaO_2 that was statistically significant ($p < .01$). In Protocol B, three room air hyperinflations at 1.5 times tidal volume produced a mean decrease in PaO_2 of 13 mm Hg. Protocol C with 15 sec of hyperinflation at 1.5 times tidal volume at 100% oxygen delivered by a Laerdal MRB, produced a mean increase in PaO_2 of 314 mm Hg that was statistically significant ($p < .01$). Conclusions regarding the efficacy of the ventilator versus the MRB for delivery of the hyperinflation breaths on postsuctioning hypoxemia cannot be made, as the ventilator breaths were at room air (21% oxygen) and the Laerdal bag was at 100% oxygen, which was not documented by an oxygen analyzer. Unlike adult endotracheal suctioning procedures, suctioning in the neonate seldom includes the component of hyperinflation. Adult lungs have a resiliency to withstand hyperinflation, whereas the premature infant's alveoli are prone to rupture. The use of hyperinflation with ETS was explored in newborns in a descriptive study by Brandstater and Muallem (1969), whose sample consisted of six term newborns, aged 7 to 34 days, treated with muscle relaxants for tetanus neonatorum. The suctioning procedure included administration of 2 ml of normal saline, hyperinflation to 25 cm H_2O, and the use of a 5 Fr. or 8 Fr. suction catheter with suction applied continuously for 4 sec. Tidal volumes decreased by 25 to 75% of control levels. Pulmonary compliance could be restored with inflation pressures of 25 to 30 cm H_2O, thus bringing attention to the magnitude of atelectasis with suctioning. The extension of their findings to the premature infant is limited because of the relative maturity and healthy state of the respiratory system in the newborns in their study as compared to the premature infant.

Adapters

Endotracheal tubes normally have an adapter or connector at the proximal end to allow for connection of the tube to the mechanical ventilator. In the 1970s a modified endotracheal tube adapter was designed with openings on the sides or end to allow the suction catheter to be introduced into the trachea without removing the patient from the ventilator. The modified endotracheal tube adapter maintains a closed airway system permitting uninterrupted ventilation, oxygenation, and positive end-expiratory pressure (PEEP) during endotracheal suctioning. Although not disconnected from the ventilator, the patient does not receive the full inspiratory pressure and end-expiratory pressure because some of the respiratory cycle pressure escapes around the catheter and through the opening in the adapter. Theoretically, if the patient remains on mechanical ventilation receiving oxygen-rich breaths and PEEP is maintained, hypoxemia can be minimized. A drawback of on-ventilator closed-system suctioning using the modified endotracheal tube adapter is the generation of intraairway negative pressure, which can result in atelectasis and alveolar collapse. Large negative intraairway pressures conceivably can be generated when the flow of gas from the ventilator is less than or equal to the flow of negative pressure with ETS.

Belling, Kelley, and Simon (1978) examined the effectiveness of a swivel adapter with a capped aperture on PaO_2 levels in 20 adult patients after open-heart surgery. Each subject was at an FIO_2 of .60, with only two subjects on 5 cm of PEEP. Each subject was exposed randomly to either disconnection from the ventilator followed by suctioning or suctioning through the adapter with 2 hours intervening between the experiments. None of the subjects received preoxygenation either by ventilator or MRB. With both suctioning methods, the endotracheal tube cuff was deflated during ETS. Arterial blood gases were drawn prior to and after each suctioning procedure, although the timing was not specified. With either suctioning method there was a statistically significant drop in pH and PaO_2 with a significant rise in $PaCO_2$. During suctioning off the ventilator, the PaO_2 dropped by $67.4 \pm 10.1\%$, with a range of 44.8 to 79.5 percent. Suctioning on the ventilator using the adapter resulted in a $24.6 \pm 10.3\%$ decline in PaO_2, with a range of 2.8 to 42.6 percent, a change that was significantly less ($p < .001$) than without the adapter. The significant decrease in PaO_2 observed with both techniques can be attributed to the lack of preoxygenation, a factor that limits the results of this study. It should be noted that there were wide ranges in the postsuctioning PaO_2 percentages, indicating that patient response to either technique was variable.

Bodai (1982) compared conventional off-ventilator suctioning to on-ventilator ETS using the adapter in seven patients with severe respiratory failure. All of the subjects had documented hypoxemia and cardiac arrhythmias with conventional suctioning. Conventional suctioning was defined as ventilator disconnection, instillation of 1 cc normal saline followed by three preoxygenation breaths delivered by an MRB at an oxygen flow rate of 15 L/min. The oxygen concentration was not verified or stated. Each catheter pass was preceded by "vigorous bagging," which was not defined. On-ventilator suctioning consisted of three ventilator "sigh" breaths without altering the percent inspired oxygen or tidal volume. The subjects' set FIO_2 ranged from .40 to 1.0, and PEEP varied from 8 to 20 cm H_2O. The two techniques were tested randomly at 2-hour intervals. Conventional suctioning resulted in a statistically significant ($p < .001$) decline in mean PaO_2 of 34.5 ± 2.7 mm Hg compared to on-ventilator suctioning of 7.0 ± 0.6 mm Hg. The investigator concluded that on-ventilator ETS using the adapter reduced ETS-induced hypoxemia because of the maintenance of PEEP and functional residual capacity, thereby preventing collapse of distal airways and alveoli. The study results must be viewed in light of the fact that the concentration of oxygen using the MRB was not monitored with a calibrated oxygen analyzer and the number and volume of "vigorous" breaths were not stated. It is conceivable that the MRB was not delivering a similar level of oxygen to permit a valid comparison; yet this is common clinical practice.

A similar investigation comparing off-ventilator suctioning to on-ventilator suctioning using the modified endotracheal tube adapter was performed by Jung and Newman (1982). Eighteen patients with acute respiratory failure who were on the Bennett MA-1 ventilator, modified to deliver intermittent mandatory ventilation (IMV) and set to one half the normal spontaneous breathing rate, participated in the study. Five of the 18 subjects had PEEP set at 10 to 12 cm H_2O, and all subjects were on an FIO_2 of greater than 0.40. The subjects were exposed randomly to either off-ventilator suctioning without pre- or posthyperoxygenation or to on-ventilator suctioning with no change in ventilator settings. After the subject's oxygen saturation and heart rate returned to baseline levels or stability had been maintained for 5 min, the subject was exposed to the alternate technique. The mean fall in arterial oxygen saturation with off-ventilator ETS was 5.55%, compared to 2.27% with on-ventilator suctioning ($p < .01$). A similar favorable response was seen in the five subjects who were receiving PEEP. The traditional disconnect method resulted in a mean decrease in SaO_2 of 12.6%, whereas the decline was only 6.2% with on-ventilator suctioning ($p < .05$). Seven of the 18 subjects with off-ventilator suctioning and 6 of the 18 with on-ventilator suctioning developed arterial oxygen saturations below 90% following ETS; these results the investigators considered unacceptable, and they recommended that hyperoxygenation would have been beneficial regardless of the method. The investigators noted that they had encountered no instances in which an intraairway negative pressure sufficient to trigger the ventilator was generated with on-ventilator closed-system suctioning.

Brown, Standbury, Merrill, Linden, and Light (1983) compared off-ventilator to on-ventilator suctioning in 22 subjects with chronic obstructive lung disease who were ventilated on the Bennett MA-1 ventilator with an IMV mode supplied from a 3 L reservoir bag. All subjects were evaluated at an FIO_2 of 0.6. Phase I of the study, off-ventilator ETS without extra breaths, resulted in a significant drop in mean SaO_2 from $94.3 \pm 2.6\%$ before ETS to $90.8 \pm 3.25\%$ after suctioning ($p < .001$). Off-ventilator ETS with presuction and postsuction breaths and on-ventilator ETS resulted in significant ($p < .005$) desaturation with all three methods. However, the mean desaturation of 1.3% with on-ventilator ETS was significantly less ($p < .05$) than the other three methods. The investigators concluded that on-ventilator ETS reduced the desaturation and shortened the recovery time. Phase II consisted of four methods randomly tested: (a) on-ventilator ETS without extra breaths or changes in ventilator settings; (b) off-ventilator ETS with six presuctioning breaths at an FIO_2 of 1.0; (c) off-ventilator ETS with six postsuctioning breaths at an FIO_2 of 1.0; (d) off-ventilator ETS with six pre- and postsuctioning breaths at FIO_2 of 1.0. The administration of six breaths at an FIO_2 of 1.0 either pre- or postsuctioning or both with off-ventilator ETS resulted in a mean desaturation that was not significantly greater than that during on-ventilator ETS. The investigators concluded that the four maneuvers designed to attenuate the desaturation associated with ETS appeared to be equivalent. The on-ventilator method showed a trend toward the lowest desaturation and the shortest recovery time of the four methods. Phase III consisted of a series of four successive 15-sec suctioning passes using two methods: (a) off-ventilator ETS with six presuctioning breaths at an FIO_2 of 1.0 and before each successive pass and after the fourth and final pass for a total of 30 breaths; and (b) on-ventilator ETS with no change in ventilator settings. Removal of the ventilator with extra breaths at an FIO_2 of 1.0 resulted in an increase in mean SaO_2 to 95.4%, which was not significant, whereas on-ventilator SaO_2 was unchanged from baseline prior to ETS. The investigators concluded that on-ventilator ETS is as effective as the currently recommended procedure of preoxygenation between each suction pass at an FIO_2 of 1.0 with off-ventilator ETS. None of the subjects in this study was on PEEP. The investigators concluded by cautioning that on-ventilator ETS should not be used with controlled or assisted ventilation without IMV because suction flow rates easily could exceed ventilator minute volume and generate large negative airway pressure or rapid cycling of the ventilator.

Baker, Baker, and Koen (1983) examined the effects of four different methods of ETS on six hypoxemic patients. Hypoxemic subjects were defined as those who required an FIO_2 of at least 0.40 and PEEP greater than 5 cm H_2O to maintain a PaO_2 greater than 60 mm Hg. All subjects were supported by IMV at rates of 6 to 10 breaths/min. The control procedure and the four methods of ETS were tested randomly. The control procedure consisted of 1 min of hyperoxygenation by raising the FIO_2 to 1.0. The cap to the swivel adapter was removed for 15 sec and no ETS was performed. Immediately following the sham, the subject was hyperoxygenated again for 1 min. Method I was the same as control, except that suctioning was performed for 15 sec through the uncapped adapter. Method II was the same as I, except that hyperinflation at two times tidal volume was performed using the ventilator during hyperoxygenation. The number of hyperinflation breaths was not stated. Method III was the same as I, except that the ventilator was replaced by an Airbird MRB with reservoir at 15 L/min oxygen and PEEP at the same level as the subject ventilator. The cap of the swivel adapter was removed to admit the catheter. Method IV was the same as III except that the adapter was removed and the suction catheter was inserted directly into the airway. Baker et al. (1983) found that the ventilator methods, I and II, were more effective than the MRB techniques (Methods III & IV) based on PaO_2 levels before, during, and after ETS ($p < .05$). The addition of hyperinflation (Method II) did not increase PaO_2 significantly when compared to Method I. The volumes delivered using the MRB were significantly less ($p < .02$) than the ventilator, suggesting that the use of the MRB results in hypoventilation. Subjects with a low IMV rate had a greater drop in PaO_2 with Method IV when the swivel adapter was not used. The decline in PaO_2 was correlated closely ($r = .90$) with the IMV rate. However, a definition of *low* IMV rate was not given in the study.

The first report of endotracheal suctioning using an adapter in neonates was an experimental study in which the cardiopulmonary effects during and following ETS were investigated (Cabal et al., 1979). Eight preterm infants with RDS received endotracheal suctioning through an adapter with side-port openings to determine the effects on heart rate and intraarterial blood oxygen saturation. The first procedure consisted of disconnection from the ventilator and intermittent positive pressure ventilation (IPPV) given by MRB for 15 sec before and after suctioning. In the second procedure the infant was suctioned through the adapter without preoxygenation. The suctioning procedure was defined as insertion of the suction catheter, instillation of .5 ml of saline, and suction applied for 5 sec.

The suctioning episodes, 128 pairs of observations, revealed a significantly lower heart rate with suctioning using the MRB than with the adapter, even though the mean baseline heart rate was higher when the MRB was used compared to the baseline heart rate with the adapter. Baseline oxygen saturation levels were similar using either method of suctioning, but the peak drop in oxygen saturation was of a greater magnitude when the MRB was used. The investigators concluded that the use of the adapter during suctioning eliminated the need for preoxygenation.

Using the same model of adapter as Cabal et al. (1979), Zmora and Merritt (1980) compared the effectiveness of suctioning through the adapter versus suctioning off-ventilator in 13 preterm and term neonates. The suctioning procedure consisted of instilling 0.2 to 0.5 ml of normal saline as irrigant, followed by 20 sec of ventilation using the MRB and then suctioning with the head turned alternately to the right and left. Between each suction pass the infant was hand-ventilated for 20 sec. This procedure was repeated for a total of four insertions of the suction catheter for each suctioning episode. The same procedure was repeated with conventional off-ventilator ETS. The investigators noted significantly less decline in $tcPO_2$ values with use of the adapter. When mean airway pressure (MAP) was calculated, it was determined that the decrease in $tcPO_2$ was related linearly to the decline in MAP. Use of the adapter resulted in low MAP, whereas conventional disconnect ETS resulted in an MAP of zero. In this study the investigators used an unusually long suctioning procedure (four suction repetitions), did not assign the order of the independent variables randomly, and did not monitor $tcPO_2$ postsuctioning to determine if there were postsuctioning differences in the $tcPO_2$ levels.

More recently, Gunderson, McPhee, and Donovan (1986), using a randomized crossover design, studied the effects of endotracheal suctioning through an adapter on $tcPO_2$ and heart rate in 11 premature infants during their first 4 days of life. Each infant was studied during three separate 2-hour periods; during each period the procedure consisted of suctioning through the adapter (partially ventilated endotracheal suction, PVETS) and suctioning with the infant removed from the ventilator (nonventilated endotracheal suction, NVETS). The order of PVETS and NVETS was randomized. The suctioning procedure consisted of no change in the inspired oxygen, rotating the infant's head to the right or left, passing the catheter until resistance was met and then withdrawing the catheter .5 cm, and applying negative pressure. The infant then was reconnected to the ventilator for 5 to 10 sec followed by the procedure repeated with the infant's head turned to the opposite side.

There were significant decreases in $tcPO_2$ during NVETS ($p < .001$) when compared to PVETS. Both the incidence and severity of hypoxic events were decreased with PVETS when compared to NVETS. Although there were no significant differences in the incidence of bradycardiac episodes related to suctioning methods, bradycardia was characterized by sudden decelerations followed by rapid recovery. The investigators noted that the temporal relationship between insertion of the suction catheter and the peak change in heart rate are evidence that bradycardia during endotracheal suctioning might be caused by the catheter stimulating the vagus nerve by mucosal stimulation. Thus, the bradycardiac episodes may be independent of levels of oxygenation. The investigators concluded that the use of an adapter significantly reduces both the incidence and severity of hypoxia during suctioning of premature infants.

SUMMARY AND FUTURE DIRECTIONS

The literature on techniques to minimize the hypoxemia associated with endotracheal suctioning reveals considerable variability in the methods employed, ranging from hyperoxygenation, hyperoxygenation/hyperventilation, and hyperoxygenation/hyperinflation to the use of the modified endotracheal tube adapter. The levels of hyperoxygenation have ranged experimentally from 10 to 20% above baseline to 100%. Whereas hyperoxygenation has been shown experimentally to minimize ETS-induced hypoxemia, the optimal level of hyperoxygenation based on the subject's baseline PaO_2 levels has not been determined. Investigations to examine known pulmonary physiologic variables that could be used to predict a subject's response to hyperoxygenation are needed. The effects of hyperoxygenation in the adult subject have not been addressed in relation to potential reabsorption atelectasis and the consequences of rapid PaO_2 changes in chronic obstructive lung disease patients whose respiratory drive is dependent upon low oxygen levels.

Hyperoxygenation/hyperventilation has been examined most extensively in newborns. The majority of the studies were not well controlled, or the suctioning procedures were not detailed sufficiently to permit a thorough evaluation or replication. The number of hyperventilation breaths often was not stated. Hyperoxygenation/hyperventilation has been shown to maintain SaO_2 levels at or above baseline; however, the extent of the oxygen elevation using oxygen saturation cannot be determined by this technique. Whereas the oxygen levels were monitored noninvasively, changes in $PaCO_2$ and pH as a consequence of hyperventilation were not studied. Well-controlled studies in newborns of similar weight and level of maturity are needed before conclusions can be drawn.

Hyperoxygenation/hyperinflation has been examined extensively in adults. The technique of administering lung hyperinflations has varied from one to three lung hyperinflations to 3 min of hyperinflations using either a manual resuscitation bag or a ventilator. In these studies little to no control was exerted over the volume of the lung hyperinflation delivered. The method of delivery of the hyperinflation breaths either via the manual resuscitation bag or ventilator has confounded the results. Well-controlled studies comparing the MRB to the ventilator as the mode of hyperinflation delivery are needed. The effect of lung hyperinflation on cardiopulmonary hemodynamics has not been examined.

The modified endotracheal tube adapter, which permits ventilation and the maintenance of PEEP and PIP during ETS, shows great promise as a technique to minimize hypoxemia in adults and newborns. However, studies to monitor the level of negative airway pressure developed with on-ventilator ETS and the consequent atelectasis must be performed to permit a complete evaluation of the technique.

The subjects in which these techniques have been tested frequently have been convenience samples of postsurgical patients with minimal respiratory complications. Well-controlled studies in subjects with varying levels of respiratory failure are needed for demonstrating which techniques are most useful. Newborns are not small adults, nor are they small children; yet despite this, many of the recommendations for endotracheal suction were taken from the adult or pediatric literature. It is recommended that future investigators examine the effect of level of maturity, age, and pathophysiological processes in relation to the subject's responses to the techniques to relieve the hypoxemia associated with endotracheal suctioning.

REFERENCES

Adlkofer, Sr. R. M., & Powaser, M. M. (1978). The effect of endotracheal suctioning on arterial blood gases in patients after cardiac surgery. *Heart & Lung, 7,* 1011–1014.

Baker, P. O., Baker, J. M., & Koen, P. A. (1983). Endotracheal suctioning techniques in hypoxemic patients. *Respiratory Care, 28,* 1563–1568.

Baun, M. M., & Flones, M. J. (1984). Cumulative effects of three sequential endotracheal suctioning episodes in the dog model. *Heart & Lung, 13,* 148–154.

Belling, D., Kelley, R. R., & Simon, R. (1978). Use of the swivel adaptor during suctioning to prevent hypoxemia in the mechanically ventilated patient. *Heart & Lung, 7,* 320–322.

Berman, I. R., & Stahl, W. M. (1968). Prevention of hypoxic complication during endotracheal suctioning. *Surgery, 63,* 586–587.

Boba, A., Cincotti, J. J., Piazza, T. E., & Landmesser, C. M. (1959). The effects of apnea, endotracheal suction, and oxygen insufflation alone and in combination, upon arterial oxygen saturation in anesthetized patients. *Journal of Laboratory and Clinical Medicine, 53,* 680–685.

Bodai, B. I. (1982). A means of suctioning without cardiopulmonary depression. *Heart & Lung, 11,* 172–176.

Bodai, B. T., Walton, C. B., Briggs, S., & Goldstein, M. (1987). A clinical evaluation of an oxygen insufflation/suction catheter. *Heart & Lung, 16,* 39–46.

Boutros, A. R. (1970). Arterial blood oxygenation during and after endotracheal suctioning in the apneic patient. *Anesthesiology, 32,* 114–118.

Brandstater, B. F., & Muallem, M. (1969). Atelectasis following tracheal suction in infants. *Anesthesiology, 31,* 468–472.

Brown, S., Standbury, D. W., Merrill, E. J., Linden, G. S., & Light, R. W. (1983). Prevention of suctioning-related arterial oxygen desaturation comparison of off-ventilator and on-ventilator suctioning. *Chest, 83,* 621, 627.

Cabal, L., Devaskar, S., Siassi, B., Plajstek, C., Waffarn, F., Blanco, C., & Hodgman, J. (1979). New endotracheal tube adaptor reducing cardiopulmonary effects of suctioning. *Critical Care Medicine, 7,* 552–555.

Criley, J. M., Blaufuss, A. H., & Kissel, G. L. (1976). Cough-induced cardiac compression. Self-administered form of cardiopulmonary resuscitation. *Journal of the American Medical Association, 236,* 1246–1250.

Cunningham, M. L., Baun, M., & Nelson, R. (1983). The effects of inflation with two levels of supplemental oxygen during endotracheal suctioning of the premature neonate. *Pediatric Research, 17,* 310. (Abstract No. 1340)

Downes, J. J., Wilson, J. F., & Goodson, D. (1961). Apnea, suction, and hyperventilation: Effect on arterial oxygen saturation. *Anesthesiology, 22,* 29–33.

Ehrhart, I. C., Hofman, W. F., & Loveland, S. R. (1981). Effects of endotracheal suction versus apnea during interruption of intermittent or continuous positive pressure ventilation. *Critical Care Medicine, 9,* 464–468.

Fanconi, S., & Duc, G. (1987). Intratracheal suctioning in sick preterm infants: Prevention on intracranial hypertension and cerebral hypoperfusion by muscle paralysis. *Pediatrics, 79,* 538–543.

Fell, T., & Cheney, F. W. (1971). Prevention of hypoxia during endotracheal suction. *Annals of Surgery, 174,* 24–28.

Fiske, G., & Baker, W. (1975). Mucosal changes in the trachea and main bronchi of newborn infants after naso-tracheal intubation. *Anesthesia Intensive Care, 3,* 209.

Fox, W. W., Morray, J. P., & Martin, R. J. (1987). Chronic neonatal lung disease. In A. A. Fanaroff & R. J. Martin (Eds.), *Neonatal-Perinatal Medicine* (pp. 628–638). St. Louis, MO: Mosby.

Goodnough, S. K. (1985). The effects of oxygen and hyperinflation on arterial oxygen tension after endotracheal suctioning. *Heart & Lung, 14*, 11–17.

Gunderson, L. P., McPhee, A. J., & Donovan, E. F. (1986). Partially ventilated endotracheal suction. *American Journal of Diseases in Children, 140*, 462–465.

Jung, R. C., & Newman, J. (1982). Minimizing hypoxia during endotracheal airway care. *Heart & Lung, 11*, 208–212.

Kergin, F. G., Bean, D. M., & Paul, W. (1948). Anoxia during intrathoracic operations: A preliminary report. *The Journal of Thoracic Surgery, 17*, 709–711.

Langrehr, E. A., Washburn, S. C., & Guthrie, M. P. (1981). Oxygen insufflation during endotracheal suctioning. *Heart & Lung, 10*, 1028–1036.

Marx, G. F., Steen, S. N., Arkins, R. E., Foster, E. S., Joffe, S., Kepes, E. R., & Schapira, M. (1968). Endotracheal suction and death. *New York State Journal of Medicine, 68*, 565–566.

Naigow, D., & Powaser, M. M. (1977). The effect of different endotracheal suction procedures on arterial blood gases in a controlled experimental model. *Heart & Lung, 6*, 808–816.

Norris, S., Campbell, L. A., & Brenkert, S. (1982). Nursing procedures and alterations in transcutaneous oxygen tension in premature infants. *Nursing Research, 31*, 330–336.

Parsons, L. C., & Shogan, J. S. O. (1984). The effects of the endotracheal tube suctioning/manual hyperventilation procedure on patients with severe closed head injuries. *Heart & Lung, 13*, 372–380.

Perlman, J. M., & Volpe, J. J. (1983). Suctioning in the preterm infant: Effects on cerebral blood flow velocity, intracranial pressure, and arterial blood pressure. *Pediatrics, 72*, 329–334.

Phelps, D. L. (1987). Retinopathy of prematurity. In A. A. Fanaroff & R. J. Martin (Eds.), *Neonatal-perinatal medicine* (pp. 1232–1234). St. Louis, MO: Mosby.

Preusser, B. A. (1985). The efficiency of commercially available manual resuscitation bags. *Focus on Critical Care, 12*, 59–61.

Raval, D., Mora, A., Yeh, T. F., & Pildes, R. S. (1980, July/August). Changes in tcPO$_2$ during tracheobronchial hygiene in neonates. *Perinatology-Neonatology*, 41–44.

Riegel, B., & Forshee, T. (1985). A review and critique of the literature on preoxygenation for endotracheal suctioning. *Heart & Lung, 14*, 507–518.

Rosen, M., & Hillard, E. K. (1962). The effects of negative pressure during tracheal suction. *Anesthesia and Analgesia, 41*, 50–57.

Rudikoff, M. T., Maughan, W. L., Effron, M., Freund, P., & Weisfeldt, M. L. (1980). Mechanism of blood flow during cardiopulmonary resuscitation. *Circulation, 61*, 345–352.

Schreiner, R. L., Smith, W. L., & Gresham, E. L. (1976). Tracheal foreign body acquired during suctioning (letter to the editor). *Journal of Pediatrics, 89*, 860.

Shim, C., Fine, N., Fernandez, R., & Williams, M. H. (1969). Cardiac arrhythmias resulting from tracheal suctioning. *Annals of Internal Medicine, 71*, 1149–1153.

Simbruner, G., Coradello, H., Fodor, M., Havelec, L., Lubec, G., & Pollak, A. (1981). Effect of tracheal suction on oxygenation, circulation, and lung mechanics in newborn infants. *Archives of Disease in Childhood, 56,* 326–330.

Skelley, B. F., Deeren, S. M., & Powaser, M. M. (1980). The effectiveness of two preoxygenation methods to prevent endotracheal suction-induced hypoxemia. *Heart & Lung, 9,* 316–323.

Stavis, R. L., & Krauss, A. N. (1980). Complications of neonatal intensive care. *Clinics in Perinatology, 7,* 107.

Storm, W. (1980). Transient bacteremia following endotracheal suctioning in ventilated newborns. *Pediatrics, 65,* 487–490.

Urban, B. J., & Weitzner, S. W. (1969). Avoidance of hypoxemia during endotracheal suction. *Anesthesiology, 31,* 473–475.

Walters, P., & Hartwig, R. (1979). Suctioning. In D. L. Levin, F. C. Morriss & G. C. Moore (Eds.), (pp. 404–408). *A practical guide to pediatric intensive care.* St. Louis, MO: Mosby.

Widdicombe, J. G. (1954). Respiratory reflexes from the trachea and bronchi of the cat. *Journal of Physiology, 123,* 55.

Zmora, E., & Merritt, T. A. (1980). Use of side-hole endotracheal tube adapter for aspiration. *American Journal of Disease in Children, 134,* 250–254.

Chapter 3

Physiological Responses to Stress

WILLA M. DOSWELL
OFFICE OF CORPORATE NURSING SERVICES
NEW YORK CITY HEALTH AND HOSPITALS CORPORATION

CONTENTS

Stress is proposed to be a major factor in the development of many illnesses such as hypertension, heart disease, and cancer, yet there is only modest empirical support to document the physiological linkages demonstrating how stress impacts these major health problems. This chapter provides a review of specific nursing research over the past decade on physiologic responses to stress. Directions for future research in this area are included. Some direction is proposed for the study of additional variables suggested by established researchers in the fields of psychology, behavioral medicine, and psychophysiology. The reader is referred to Elliott and Eisdorfer (1982) and Goldberger and Breznitz (1982), who present comprehensive reviews of the state of the art of stress research in behavioral medicine and psychology. Because of the interdisciplinary nature of the study of stress, it is

51

appropriate that the insights and recommendations of researchers from these fields be incorporated into future research.

METHODS OF RETRIEVAL

This chapter was limited to a review of nursing research published from 1977 through 1987. Studies reviewed included those in which investigators: (a) dealt with any age group and clinical specialty in which stress was a variable coupled with a dependent physiologic variable; (b) used the term stress in the study title or problem statement; or (c) included stress in the theoretical framework. Only studies conducted in the United States were included. Studies of animal subjects were not reviewed. Quantitative analysis methods were not used in reviewing studies because of the small samples and dissimilar nature of the studies comprising the research.

A DIALOG computer search of the *Cumulative Index to Nursing and Allied Health Literature* (CINAHL) was used, covering the period of 1983 to 1987. A manual search of CINAHL was conducted to retrieve studies published during the period 1977 through 1982. Identified were 18 studies that met the criteria for this review. Relevant studies were retrieved, and data about study variables, sample size and characteristics, measurement tools, study design, statistical tests, p levels, and test values were placed on coding sheets as recommended by Cooper (1984).

Additionally, a DIALOG search was made of the nursing subfile of MEDLINE for the same time period to identify additional references not included in CINAHL. No additional studies were retrieved.

A sample of 350 references, 1977 to 1987, of the DIALOG Psych-INFO subfile on stress reactions ($N = 1500$) was searched for nurse authorship, resulting in only one relevant reference. The inability to search DIALOG for authorship by professional field prevented the search of the entire PsychINFO subfiles on stress reactions/physiological correlates. All literature searches and retrieval were completed by the author.

A review of the bibliographies by other authors (Fagin, 1987; Hefferin, 1980; Kim, 1987; Lindsey, 1982, 1983; Lowery, 1987; Lyon & Werner, 1987; Pollock, 1984) who have compiled reviews of stress and/or physiologic response research in nursing also was included in the search. Some bibliographic entries (Bargagliotti & Trygstad, 1987;

Singer, 1985; Sparacino, 1982; Wolf, Wolf, & Hare, 1950; Wolman, 1973) have been included in the references at the end of the chapter as sources of in-depth review of certain aspects and methodologies of stress research.

PHYSIOLOGICAL STRESS RESPONSES

The 19 nursing studies on physiologic responses to stress were divided into four subject categories: life events; vocal stress; hospital–environmental stressors; and miscellaneous, covering single studies. Seven studies were published from 1977 through 1979, and 11 studies were published from 1980 through 1987. A majority of the physiological response variables examined in these studies were cardiovascular. Ages of the samples in these studies ranged from 18 to 74 years, with a mean age of 40. Sample sizes ranged from a low of 5 to a high of 200 ($M = 45$). The majority of investigators had both males and females in their samples, did not include subjects' ethnicity, and tended to report modestly statistically significant results. The method of sample recruitment was not reported routinely.

In a comprehensive review of a decade of physiological phenomena in research in critical care nursing, Lindsey (1984) concluded that the studies on physiological phenomena were so diverse and fragmented that limited contributions were added to nursing's knowledge base. Lowery (1987) concluded that nurses had not examined the major theoretical and methodologic issues of stress research but instead adapted a theoretical framework, a tool, and a physiological variable without careful articulation of their relevance to the nursing phenomena under study. For this review physiologic responses are defined as mechanisms of physical functioning in health and functional responses in illness (Kim, 1987).

In a review of research on physiological responses in health and illness, Kim (1987) stated that nurse physiologists primarily have examined cellular, pathological, and microbiological responses, which has been important research but not readily applicable to patient care. More relevant to nursing practice would be the physical illnesses documented in the literature as influenced by stress. These illnesses included colds, minor infections, bronchial asthma, peptic ulcer, hypertension, cancer, hyperthyroidism, and sudden cardiac death.

Any discussion of nursing research on physiological responses to stress must be governed by several points. First, for the most part there are single studies with occasional study couplets examining the same variable; thus, the findings do not provide a substantive base for application to practice. Second, given that research results always are probabilistic, the findings of any one or even two studies of a particular variable may have occurred simply by chance and, therefore, are not necessarily applicable to practice. Third, the published nursing research on physiologic responses to stress may be small because there is a tendency for investigators not to submit studies with nonsignificant findings for publication, or for some journals not to accept such studies for publication.

For the relationship between variables tested in research to have significance for the advancement of knowledge, the investigator needs both to show statistical significance and to demonstrate how much of a difference was present. The strength of the relationship is just as important as whether the relationship between variables reaches statistical significance (Cooper, 1984). For the most part, reports of the studies did not contain enough information or data to look at the strength of the relationship and the effect size.

Life Events

Haughey, Brasure, Maloney, and Saxon (1984) examined the relation between major and daily life events and cardiac arrhythmias in a sample ($N = 100$) of men and women aged 18 to 74 years with cardiac disease. The sample was not matched with a control group by diagnosis and therapeutic plan. Cardiac arrhythmias were monitored by Holter monitor. Study results were nonsignificant for the relationship between major life events during the previous year, as measured by the Holmes and Rahe Social Readjustment Rating Scale (1967) and physiological responses. There was a small significant correlation between sinus tachycardia and daily stressors occurring within the 24 hours before the patient was monitored. Gender differences were not reported. The findings of a negative correlation between social interaction and a decrease in cardiac arrhythmias held interesting possibilities for future research in view of current hospital policies regarding patient visiting.

Like Woods, Most, and Longenecker (1985), Haughey et al. (1984) relied on a personal diary for monitoring daily stressors. A second measure such as Delongis' shortened version of the Hassles Scale (Delongis, Coyne, Dakof, Folkman, & Lazarus, 1982) might have been a useful concurrent measure. An explicit theoretical framework of stress was not delineated in the study. Haughey et al. suggested replication of the study with a larger sample.

Woods et al. (1985) were among the first investigators to study major and daily life stressors in females experiencing premenstrual symptoms. The investigators utilized the concept of hassles, the day-to-day repetitive problems and irritations many individuals encounter. This concept was derived from the work of Lazarus and Folkman (1984). The study was exploratory and had no explicit guiding theoretical framework to explain the variable linkages. Study findings showed a modest positive correlation between daily stressors and increased premenstrual symptoms. An opportunity to provide additional data on the Hassles Scale (Kanner, Coyne, Schaefer, & Lazarus, 1981) was missed by using a diary to measure daily stressors in this study. Instead, a self-report assessment of physiological responses was used. A suggestion for further research would be to replicate the study using the Hassles Scale and employ an endocrine measure for the physiological variable.

Murphy (1984) investigated the daily stressors and effect on health of individuals who experienced personal or property loss in a natural disaster. The sample of males and females ($N = 63$), with a mean age of 42 years, completed the Sarason, Johnson, and Siegel Life Experiences Survey (1978), the Hassles Scale, and a self-report of physiologic responses. The study's conceptual framework was based on Lazarus' conceptual model of stress (1981). The findings revealed that subjects across four disaster groups and a control group were not significantly different from each other in the amount of stress experienced 11 months after the disaster. The four disaster groups reported more life events but fewer numbers of hassles than the control group.

Though interesting, Murphy's (1984) study demonstrated a major weakness of field research, which was a lack of control over extraneous variables and events and a reliance on the subjects' recall of stressful events almost 1 year later. A larger matched sample and a tool more representative of life events should be included in a similar study.

Thomas and Groer (1986) conducted the only study reviewed with children as subjects. The purpose was to examine the relationship of selected anthropomorphic (height, weight, body mass), demographic, lifestyle, and stress variables on the blood pressure of rural, urban, and suburban adolescents. A life events questionnaire designed for adolescents was used. A random zero sphygmomanometer was used for the measurement of blood pressure. This sphygmomanometer operated similarly to a conventional one except that an adjustment to an undisclosed zero level was done prior to each measure to reduce observer bias.

Stressors reported most frequently were hassles with parents, hassles with siblings, and making new friends. Females had more stressors than males, although males had higher blood pressure. Using multiple regression procedures, urban residence was the strongest predictor of female systolic pressure. Future research needs to be designed to demonstrate the stressor–blood pressure linkages more directly.

A study of the relationship between Type A or B behavior, life satisfaction, interpersonal trust, and blood pressure was conducted by Johnson et al. (1987), who found a low, significant correlation between these psychosocial variables and blood pressure. The study report contained a description of the reliability and validity testing done for the Risk Factor Questionnaire, which was developed by the investigators and used to measure the three psychosocial variables. The study was based on the Selye (1983) theory of stress, but the investigators provided no explanation of the theoretical linkages between study variables. They utilized a nonspecific response theory of stress to describe transactional stress variables.

Life events research has been a popular area of stress research, but the findings correlate only modestly with physiologic response outcomes. Research to explain proposed stress/physiological response linkages is lacking; yet as Lowery (1987) has pointed out, it is the study of these proposed linkages that might have the most impact on nursing care of patients in stressful situations. One difficulty in correlating life events with physiologic responses is that the change in the physiologic responses may be associated with the illness or treatment variables and not the preceding life event.

Vocal Stress

Sparacino, Hansell, and Smyth (1979) examined speech behaviors observed during interviews and blood pressure correlates of Type A personality in black, urban females. The findings were that Type A explosive loud speech did not correlate significantly with increased blood pressure. The original purpose of the study, to explore mediating mechanisms linking Type A behavior and coronary heart disease, could not be determined with the correlational design that was used. Suggested areas for future investigations included expanding the physiological variables explored to include telemetry, biochemical physiological variables, and an examination of speech in a more naturalistic setting.

Brockway (1979) studied vocal responses to structured (artificial) and naturally occurring stressors. Instead of using the voice characteristics monitored by Sparacino et al. (1979), Brockway employed the psychological stress evaluator (PSE), an instrument that detects, measures, and graphically displays stress-related components of the human voice. The term PSE is something of a misnomer because physiological microtremors of voice musculature actually were monitored, from which the psychological state of stress was inferred.

In Brockway's (1979) study a sample of nursing students ($N = 17$) was divided into experimental and control groups, and interviewed twice. The experimental group was interviewed before and after a major examination. The control group was tested two days following the examination period and again eight days later. Although statistically significant differences were found between the two groups, the study needed replication in a larger sample because the sample size limited the generalizability of findings. Additionally, a conceptual framework should be developed in which stress, as opposed to anxiety, and theoretical linkages with physiological vocal responses are defined.

Hurley (1983) also selected vocal response as the dependent variable in a study on marital conflict. Hurley defined stress according to the standard psychosomatic definition but did not identify an explicit theoretical framework linking the study variables. Hurley hypothesized a positive correlation between a stressful interaction and stress patterning as demonstrated by vocal stress analysis, using the PSE, and found no support for any of the hypothesized relationships. She concluded that a single, artificially induced conflict was not an appropriate method for the measurement of vocal physiologic responses to stress.

Hospital–Environmental Stressors

B. J. Volicer and L. Volicer (1978) examined the effects of nine hospital stressors on changes in the following cardiovascular variables: heart rate, systolic and diastolic blood pressure, stroke volume, and cardiac output. The study of 463 hospitalized patients, with a mean age of 47 years, was designed using the patient record for data collection of the physiological indices. An investigator-developed paper-and-pencil tool was used to measure hospital stressors such as lack of information and threat of severe illness. The sample was divided into four groups by length of stay and severity of illness. The investigators found that two low-severity groups experiencing minor to moderate stress had corresponding changes in heart rate. In the high medical severity of illness group, only increased blood pressure was correlated with increased hospital stress. In the high surgical severity of illness group, stroke volume was correlated inversely with increased hospital stress.

The Volicers' (1978) failure to match subjects by diagnosis and the many uncontrolled variables may have contributed to the nonsignificant to modest findings. The absence of systematic measurement of the physiological variables was a major weakness of the study. In the use of change scores, there was no consideration of baseline levels prior to calculating change scores.

In four additional studies investigators examined the stressful effects of the hospital environment on physiological responses. Errico's (1977) investigation of the effects of information feedback versus no information feedback on cardiovascular variables (heart rate, blood pressure, and respirations) was designed well. The condition of no information feedback generally resulted in higher physiological responses. The stress literature was reviewed; and although a complete theoretical framework was not reported, some stress concepts were linked to provide direction for the study. Errico used a convenience sample of 18- to 40-year-old male and female volunteers ($N = 200$). This study was the only one reviewed that included a statement of the power and effect size used to compute the sample size.

Schwartz and Brenner (1979) wanted to determine the effectiveness of three nursing interventions in reducing patient stress at time of transfer from the critical care unit to a general medical unit. Physiological responses of shortness of breath, chest pain, nausea, and lightheadedness were assessed by paper-and-pencil test. Creatine phosphokinase was measured from blood samples obtained from participants.

Results indicated that both family communication and a visit by the nurse from the receiving unit contributed to a reduction in reported physiological responses to stress. The findings lack generalizability because of an unspecified theoretical framework, an imprecise definition of stress, the use of self-report measures of physiological response, and a small sample size ($N = 20$).

Fuller and Foster (1982) examined the effects of family- and friend-focused interactions versus nurse–patient task interaction on physiological responses to the presumed stress of being an intensive care unit patient. Proposing to replicate the research of Brown (1976), the study was designed to examine specific physiologic responses to stress, for example, heart rate and blood pressure. Fuller and Foster reported no significant differences in cardiovascular responses to the three types of interaction and concluded that family visits were no more stressful than a routine nurse–patient interaction or a nurse–patient task-oriented interaction. The study sample was small and unmatched for diagnosis, so the clinical implications the authors discussed seem premature. Consistent with Brown's findings, those of Fuller and Foster showed no significant increase or decrease in heart rate or blood pressure changes after family visits.

Vanson, Katz, and Krekeler (1980) also investigated the effects of hospital–environmental stressors on physiologic responses. Specifically, they examined the effect on study patients of watching a stressful procedure being performed on another patient located either in an open ward or an enclosed cubicle. The procedures observed were Swan-Ganz catheter insertion, pacemaker insertion, and cardioversion. The investigators did not specify a theoretical framework or a definition of stress. The criteria and rationale for stressor selection were not reported. The physiological variable pulse rate, measured on an electrocardiogram monitor, was computed without regard for differences in prestimulus levels. The subject selection procedure was not delineated, and the statistical analysis method was reported incompletely.

Miscellaneous Studies

A study by Guzzetta and Forsyth (1979) was included in the review because of the investigators' attempt to develop a typology of stress observed in acutely ill patients. The researchers defined stress and stressor in the tradition of Selye (1980) and psychophysiological stress as responses caused by or related to the presence of a stimulus or stressor. A conceptual framework was presented showing the relationship between type of stressor and physiological response elicited.

Guzzetta and Forsyth (1979) presented a pilot project to test the typology, though the reporting was insufficient to evaluate adequately its reliability, validity, and applicability to nursing. The investigators tested the typology on a small sample ($N = 5$) of coronary care unit patients, using an anxiety–depression scale as a measure of stress. The pilot study was conducted to develop and test the physiologic response categories and identify etiologic parameters and characteristics of stressors. Labels of low, medium, high, and extreme psychophysiological stress were identified as diagnostic categories. Results of the pilot study validated the existence of 60% of the proposed typology. Specific methods for instrument validation were not reported. The investigators recognized the need for a well-designed study to test the typology further.

Examining the effects of the stress of surgery on circadian rhythms of selected physiological responses, Farr, Keene, Samson, and Michael (1984) found greater rhythmic variation in catecholamines after the patient returned home. The literature review contained few related nursing studies, and Farr et al. did not define stress or conceptualize the variables within a stress theoretical framework. Although the investigators reported significant findings, they did not indicate how the responses might be harmful for the patient. They recommended future research, but there was no proposed theoretical linkage of stress and circadian rhythms. The size of the sample ($N = 11$) made analysis and interpretation of these data highly speculative. What is needed is a redesigned study and replication with a larger sample. Directions that Farr et al. might have suggested for future research included best times to schedule treatment regimens and activities and whether nursing interventions could enhance a return of the patient's circadian rhythms.

Only one researcher, Randolph (1984), included measurement of the physiological responses of skin conductance, skin temperature, and electromyograph responses to an environmental stressor (a motion picture film). Specifically, Randolph focused on a comparison of these physiologic responses to therapeutic or physical touch interventions. Again, a definition of stress and a theoretical framework linking stress to therapeutic touch were not delineated clearly. Skin conductance and electromyography responses were defined and monitored as baseline levels instead of as responses. The Randolph double blind design was the first study to improve significantly the research design in order to affirm the validity of therapeutic touch as an intervention. However the lack of a distinct theoretical framework linking physiological responses to stress limits the interpretation of the findings.

Guzzetta (1979) examined the effect of teaching cardiac rehabilitation to male postmyocardial infarction patients ($N = 45$) during three time periods after transfer from a coronary care unit. Urinary cortisol was the physiological variable monitored. Anxiety was defined operationally as a stress indicator and was measured by an author-developed anxiety scale. The reviewer could not find evidence in the report that the scale met criteria for instrument construction as delineated in Waltz, Strickland, and Lenz (1984). Guzzetta reported that learning was more effective if teaching was done 7 days post-CCU transfer, when patients experienced the least anxiety. Urinary cortisol levels did not differ on days 3, 7, and 11. A serendipitous finding was that 42% of the patients demonstrated abnormally low cortisol levels. There was no correlation between cortisol level and score on the anxiety scale. Further exploration of this phenomenon is warranted.

Catchpole's (1985) investigation of the stress reduction effects of receiving preoperative medications versus a 30-minute stay in a preoperative waiting area without medications prior to surgery was an important area with high applicability to nursing practice. Plasma catecholamine level was the physiological measure. Catchpole concluded that patients receiving preoperative narcotic medications had higher plasma catecholamine levels than patients receiving no preoperative medication. A paper-and-pencil measure of the patient's perception of the presence of stressors would have strengthened the study design. The lack of measurement of stressors along with the small sample size ($N = 40$) and failure to match for diagnosis or type of surgery, renders the findings of limited usefulness to practice except to invite replication.

Tallman (1982) assessed the effect of a physical stressor (vein intracatheter insertion) on glucose, insulin, and free fatty acid levels obtained in a sample of 21 normal volunteers. A control group was not included in the research design. Tallman found that subsequently drawn glucose levels were not affected by intracatheter insertion, but insulin and free fatty acid were affected. Tallman's tentative conclusions that drawing of insulin and free fatty acid levels should begin 15 to 30 minutes respectively after intracatheter insertion were clinically important but of limited generalizability without further testing. Although the stressor was identified, there was no conceptual framework linking the stressor with the physiologic responses. Based on clinical experience, the investigator presumed that the intracatheter insertion was a stressor, but no objective measure of stress was included in this study. If one subscribes to Lazarus's theory of stress, then an important component of the stress response was omitted when this objective measure of the individual's perception of the stress was not observed.

SUMMARY

Human stress research rarely has involved life-threatening or uniformly stressful situations. Thus the methods for studying its effects in humans and for defining it conceptually and operationally are not as precise as in other fields of research. The impact of stress on health can be summarized as follows: Individuals experiencing a variety of sudden disruptive or upsetting events are at increased risk for adversive outcomes, such as illness. In general, laboratory research evidence has suggested that individual reactions to stressors are associated with transient physiological changes. What those changes mean and the theoretical linkages connecting them to stress must be developed. Lyon and Werner (1987) have stated that looking at response models of stress is incompatible with nursing's view of human experiences. However, researchers building their studies on the Lazarus conceptual model (Lazarus & Folkman, 1984) of stress as a transaction between man and his environment would reduce this incompatibility substantially. This reviewer concurs with Lyon and Werner (1987) in the opinion that research of physiologic responses to stress has been linked only nominally to a conceptual framework forming the foundation for the generation of study hypotheses.

Wolman (1973) defined stress as a condition of physical or mental strain producing autonomic nervous system changes. Anxiety was defined as a reaction to internal threat, the response engendered when the threat is met in an unsatisfying way. In some of the studies reviewed, the distinction between these two concepts was blurred.

The number of published nursing studies on physiologic responses to stress has been too small and disjointed to provide exploration of a consistent set of variables. The research over the past decade included a predominance of single diverse studies measuring single cardiovascular variables, and utilizing Selye's (1983) theory of stress. The findings of these studies were generally of low to moderate statistical significance, and the methodologies were conceptualized and designed too loosely to provide definitive explanations or confirmation of physiological correlates of stress.

The research also has suffered from a confusion in conceptual definitions and theoretical frameworks related to stress that pervades many disciplines studying stress. Nurse researchers primarily employed cardiovascular physiologic responses, though there were signs of expansion as exemplified in studies on vocal stress and endocrine measures. Training in advanced physiological and biochemical theory and measurement will aid in the incorporation of other physiological variables in studies of stress.

Some investigators have failed to consider the law of initial values in their computation of physiologic responses to stress. This law states that the higher the prestimulus level of the physiological variable under study, the less response will be noted in that variable when stimulated or stressed (Wilder, 1962). Lacey (1956) has suggested that transformation of autonomic lability, the momentary displacement of level as a function of some imposed stimulus, into a score corrects for the practice of computing algebraic or percentage changes in quantifying physiological responses.

RECOMMENDATIONS FOR FUTURE RESEARCH

Future directions for nursing research on physiologic responses to stress should include the examination of daily life stressors and their influence on patient noncompliance with therapeutic regimens in such illnesses as hypertension, diabetes, and obesity. The advantages of portable and telemetric physiologic measures, such as are available for blood pressure monitoring, need to be explored. Research into the relationship between daily life events and high blood pressure may gain a boost from the recent technological advent of 24-hour automated ambulatory blood pressure recorders. Portable ambulatory recorders enable a circadian pattern to be examined and can assist researchers in pinpointing the peak, trough, and patterning of blood pressure responses to daily stressors. Monitoring of physiologic responses to daily life stressors over a period of days could be enhanced by telemetry.

There was little research on physiologic responses to stress in children. The adequacy of the infant to handle environmental stressors during the first year of life so as to interact effectively with the environment needs further study. The effect of stress on mother–infant contact, infant feeding patterns, and motor activity could be elucidated partially by the inclusion of physiological measures.

Volicer and Bohannon (1975) suggested that patient stressors, such as unfamiliar surroundings and loss of independence, be examined for the improvement of patient care. In a basic overview of research employing physiological responses, Hopping (1980) suggested the importance of patient stressors to nurse researchers and the need for researchers to be familiar with the physiology of stress and its consequences. For example, what are the biological indicators of the effectiveness of medications? What physiological responses are evident when a pain medication is administered on time as opposed to late? What are patient-specific physiological indicators of a delay in answering a hospitalized patient's call light, or being hospitalized far from home? What are physiological indicators that satisfactory preoperative teaching, counseling, and emotional support have been given to the patient prior to surgery? What are the physiological concomitants of being told about a serious illness or impending death? Or not being told what the diagnosis is? What are the physiologic responses to stress of women experiencing premenstrual syndrome? All of these areas identified are areas of stress for patients.

Hoskins's (1981) Interpersonal Conflict Scale may be coupled with physiological responses to stress in autism, other behavioral disturbances, and conditions of neurological dysfunction and developmental lag. Although not an effective single measure of physiological responses to stress, paper-and-pencil measures of a subject's perception of his body's reaction to stress might be a useful measure coupled with a measure of a physiological response.

Pollock (1984) suggested that stress researchers needed to adopt a theoretical framework that takes into account the circumstances under which the stressor occurs and the psychological characteristics and reactions of the respondent. She further recommended that research be designed to examine the specific mechanisms eliciting a stress reaction and nursing interventions to prevent or at least minimize the stressors that adversely affect health.

Selye (1980) and Lyon and Werner (1987) affirmed the recommendation that multiple physiological measures, perhaps a battery of measures yielding a stress index, were needed to monitor stress responses. The incorporation of physiological response variables into stress research designs meets this recommendation and further reduces one of the weaknesses of physiological response studies, ascribing causality to a physiological response. The research of Brockway (1979) and Hurley (1983) suggested the psychological stress evaluator is promising as one of the multiple measures of physiological responses to stress.

Hefferin (1980) asserted the need for research to identify events perceived as stressful by people at different points in the life cycle. This approach might be coupled with physiological response variables to measure the stress outcome, and longitudinal data then might contribute important information to understanding how the so-called stress illnesses evolve.

Exploring the concept of John Henryism, James, LaCroix, Kleinbaum, and Strogatz (1984) have studied the effects of psychosocial job stressors on blood pressure level of Southern workers. John Henryism is a belief that obstacles can be overcome by a combination of confronting stressors, hard work, and determination. The John Henryism scale (James et al., 1984) might be a useful measure coupled with cardiovascular variables to study stressors in executives and other workers at risk from stress from high-performance job pressures or the worker who has multiple jobs.

Singer (1985) has stated that remaining gaps in stress research include formulating theoretical frameworks linking physiological aspects with other aspects of the stress response, and studies of the influence of positive events as stressors. The new emphasis on exploring positive stressors might be carried into physiological indicators as well. What are the concurrent physiological indicators of pleasant stress? What theoretical frameworks best support these interactions? Is positive mood an effective mediator of stress? Are physiological markers sensitive indicators for demonstrating the magnitude of the stress response?

Advances in measurement of the stress hormones and metabolic products of the stress response provide researchers with an opportunity for studying a variety of biological markers that may change with the type, length, and severity of stress-related illnesses (Fagin, 1987). Such research would contribute to preventive and therapeutic nursing interventions to improve the quality of patient health.

The study of physiological responses to stress currently involves the study of biological indicators, such as the adrenal hormones and the immune system. The nurse researcher now has a wide variety of variables to study, which include adrenocorticotrophic hormone, androgen, estrogen, follicle stimulating hormone, luteinizing hormone, thyroid stimulating hormone, and growth hormone. The development of theoretical linkages between these indicators and specific stressors would be a major contribution to the field of stress research. But researchers employing these variables will have to think through carefully the theoretical frameworks linking stress variables with these biological indicators.

Peripheral cardiovascular indicators such as heart rate, blood pressure, and vasoconstriction continue to be fruitful areas for research. Another group of common physiological indicators consists of electrodermal phenomena. Selye (1983) has reaffirmed the usefulness of galvanic skin response as a physiological indicator of psychosocial stress, although it is not as sensitive a measure of stress induced by other agents. As long as the researcher is cognizant of its limitations, it should not be abandoned as one of a set of multiple measures for examining the stress response.

Antonovsky (1979) has identified a new aspect of stress research that may have relevance for nursing practice. It is the study of stress-resistant individuals, those people who do not seem to be overwhelmed by major or minor stresses. The physiology and behavior characteristics of this group have not been studied systematically. Perhaps studying the physiological and behavioral characteristics of individuals at particular risk for a major illness but who do not develop it might assist in the prevention or minimization of symptoms and pathology in those who do.

Lindsey (1982) conducted a review of physiological nursing research literature from 1970 to 1980 and concluded that the number of nursing studies employing physiological variables was small and, for the most part, not directly relevant to nursing practice. She recommended that future research be more cumulative, building in specific areas of most relevance to nurses. Longitudinal prospective studies are needed.

This reviewer concludes that studies reviewed utilized unidimensional physiologic measures when multiple measures might have provided a stronger confirmation of proposed variable relationships. Lyon and Werner's (1987) review of stress studies (Brockway, 1979; Errico, 1977; Guzzetta, 1979; Randolph, 1984; Schwartz & Brenner, 1979) presented a comprehensive discussion of threats to internal and external validity as described in Cook and Campbell (1979). Lyon and Werner (1987) stated that nurses who wish to contribute to stress research need to give more attention to reducing internal and external threats to a study's validity, to more precise measurement of stress variables based on a congruent and compatible theoretical base, and to more rigor in the statistics utilized to analyze study data.

REFERENCES

Antonovsky, K. A. (1979). *Health, stress, and coping: New perspectives on mental and physical well-being.* San Francisco: Jossey-Bass.

Bargagliotti, L. A., & Trygstad, L. N. (1987). Differences on stress and coping findings: A reflection of social realities or methodology? *Nursing Research, 36,* 170–173.

Brockway, F. (1979). Situational stress and temporal changes in self-report and vocal measurements. *Nursing Research, 28,* 20–24.

Brown, A. J. (1976). Effect of family visits on the blood pressure and heart rate of patients in CCU. *Heart and Lung, 5,* 291–296.

Catchpole, M. (1985). Do preoperative medications reduce emotional stress as measured by plasma catecholamine levels? *Journal of the American Association of Nurse Anesthetists, 53,* 327–331.

Cook, T. D., & Campbell, D. T. (1979). *Quasi-experimental design and analysis: Issues in field settings.* Chicago: Rand McNally.

Cooper, H. M. (1984). *The integrative research review: A systematic approach: Vol. 2. Applied social research methods series.* Beverly Hills: Sage.

Delongis, A., Coyne, J. C., Dakof, G., Folkman, S., & Lazarus, R. S. (1982). Relationship of daily hassles, uplifts, and major life events to health status. *Health Psychology, 1*(2), 119–136.

Elliott, G. R., & Eisdorfer, C. (Eds.). (1982). *Stress and human health: Analysis and implications of research.* New York: Springer Publishing Co.

Errico, E. (1977). Effect of cardiac monitoring on blood pressure, apical rate, and respiration with and without information feedback. *International Journal of Nursing Studies, 14,* 77–90.

Fagin, C. M. (1987). Stress: Implications for nursing research. *Image, 19,* 38–41.

Farr, L., Keene, A., Samson, D., & Michael, A. (1984). Alterations in circadian excretion of urinary variables and physiological indicators of stress following surgery. *Nursing Research, 33,* 140–146.

Fuller, B. F., & Foster, C. M. (1982). The effects of family/friend visits vs. staff interaction on stress/arousal of surgical intensive care patients. *Heart and Lung, 11,* 457–463.

Goldberger, L., & Breznitz, S. (Eds.). (1982). *Handbook of stress: Theoretical and clinical aspects.* New York: Free Press.

Guzzetta, C. E. (1979). Relationship between stress and learning. *Advances in Nursing Science, 1*(4), 35–49.

Guzzetta, C. E., & Forsyth, G. L. (1979). Nursing diagnostic pilot study: Psychophysiologic stress. *Advances in Nursing Science, 2*(1), 27–44.

Haughey, B. P., Brasure, J., Maloney, M., & Saxon, G. (1984). The relationship between stressful life events and electrocardiogram abnormalities. *Heart and Lung, 13,* 405–410.

Hefferin, E. A. (1980). Life-cycle stressors: An overview of research. *Family and Community Health, 2*(4), 71–101.

Holmes, T. H., & Rahe, R. H. (1967). The social readjustment rating scale. *Journal of Psychosomatic Research, 2,* 213–218.

Hopping, L. (1980). Physiological response to stress. A nursing concern. *Nursing Forum, 19,* 259–269.

Hoskins, C. N. (1981). Psychometrics in nursing research: Construction of an interpersonal conflict scale. *Research in Nursing and Health, 4,* 243–249.

Hurley, P. M. (1983). Communication variables and voice analysis of marital conflict stress. *Nursing Research, 32,* 164–169.

James, S., LaCroix, A., Kleinbaum, D., & Strogatz, D. (1984). John Henryism and blood pressure differences among black men. II. The role of occupational stressors. *Journal of Behavioral Medicine, 7*(3), 259–278.

Johnson, M. N., Beard, M. T., Valdez, R., Mott, J. A., Hughes, O., & Fomby, B. (1987). Psychological stress and blood pressure levels in black women. *Journal of the National Black Nurses' Association, 1*(2), 41–54.

Kanner, A. D., Coyne, C., Schaefer, C., & Lazarus, R. (1981). Comparison of two modes of stress measurement: Daily hassles and uplifts versus major life events. *Journal of Behavioral Medicine, 4*(1), 1–39.

Kim, M. J. (1987). Physiological responses in health and illness: An overview. In J. J. Fitzpatrick, R. L. Taunton, & J. A. Benoliel (Eds.), *Annual review of nursing research, Volume 5* (pp. 79–104). New York: Springer Publishing Co.

Lacey, J. I. (1956). The evaluation of autonomic responses: Toward a general solution. *Annals of the New York Academy of Sciences, 67,* 123–164.

Lazarus, R. S. (1981). Stress and coping paradigm. In C. Eisdorfer, D. Cohen, A. Kleinman, & P. Maxim (Eds.), *Models for clinical psychopathology* (pp. 177–214). New York: Spectrum.

Lazarus, R. S., & Folkman, S. (1984). *Stress, appraisal, and coping.* New York: Springer Publishing Co.

Lindsey, A. (1982). Phenomena and physiological variables of relevance to nursing. Review of a decade of work: Part I. *Western Journal of Nursing Research, 4,* 343–364.

Lindsey, A. (1983). Phenomena and physiological variables of relevance to nursing: A review of a decade of work: Part II. *Western Journal of Nursing Research, 5,* 41–63.

Lindsey, A. (1984). Research for clinical practice: Physiological phenomena. *Heart and Lung, 13,* 496–506.

Lowery, B. J. (1987). Stress research: Some theoretical and methodological issues. *Image, 19,* 42–46.

Lyon, B., & Werner, J. (1987). Ten years of practice-relevant research. In J. J. Fitzpatrick, R. L. Taunton, & J. A. Benoliel (Eds.), *Annual review of nursing research, Volume 5* (pp. 3–22). New York: Springer Publishing Co.

Murphy, S. A. (1984). Stress levels and health status of victims of a natural disaster. *Research in Nursing and Health, 7,* 205–215.

Pollock, S. E. (1984). The stress response. *Critical Care Quarterly, 6*(4), 1–14.

Randolph, G. L. (1984). Therapeutic and physical touch: Physiological response to stressful stimuli. *Nursing Research, 33,* 33–36.

Sarason, I. G., Johnson, J. H., & Siegel, J. M. (1978). Assessing the impact of life changes: Development of the Life Experiences Survey. *Journal of Consulting and Clinical Psychology, 46,* 932–946.

Schwartz, L. P., & Brenner, Z. R. (1979). Critical care unit transfer reducing patient stress through nursing interventions. *Heart and Lung, 8,* 540–545.

Selye, H. (1980). *Selye's guide to stress research* (Vol. 1). New York: Van Nostrand Reinhold.

Selye, H. (1983). *Selye's guide to stress research* (Vol. 2). New York: Van Nostrand Reinhold.

Singer, J. E. (1985). Traditions of stress research: Integrative comments. *Issues in Mental Health Nursing, 7*(1), 25–33.

Sparacino, J. (1982). Blood pressure, stress, and mental health. *Nursing Research, 31,* 89–94.
Sparacino, J., Hansell, S., & Smyth, K. (1979). Type A (Coronary-Prone) behavior and transient blood pressure change. *Nursing Research, 28,* 198–204.
Tallman, V. (1982). Effects of venipuncture on glucose, insulin, and free fatty acid levels. *Western Journal of Nursing Research, 4,* 21–30.
Thomas, S. P., & Groer, M. W. (1986). Relationship of demographic, lifestyle, and stress variables to blood pressure in adolescents. *Nursing Research, 35,* 169–172.
Vanson, Sister R. J., Katz, B. M., & Krekeler, K. (1980). Stress effects on patients in critical care units from procedures performed on others. *Heart and Lung, 9,* 494–497.
Volicer, B. J., & Bohannon, M. W. (1975). A hospital stress rating scale. *Nursing Research, 24,* 352–359.
Volicer, B. J., & Volicer, L. (1978). Cardiovascular changes associated with stress during hospitalization. *Journal of Psychosomatic Research, 22,* 159–168.
Waltz, C. F., Strickland, O. R., & Lenz, E. R. (1984). *Measurement in nursing research.* Philadelphia: F. A. Davis.
Wilder, J. (1962). The law of initial values. *Annals of New York Academy of Sciences, 98,* 1211–1220.
Wolf, H. G., Wolf, S. G., Jr., & Hare, C. C. (Eds.). (1950). *Life stress and bodily disease.* Baltimore: Williams & Wilkins.
Wolman, B. (Ed.). (1973). *Book of general psychology.* Englewood Cliffs, NJ: Prentice-Hall.
Woods, N. F., Most, A., & Longenecker, G. D. (1985). Major life events, daily stressors, and perimenstrual symptoms. *Nursing Research, 34,* 263–267.

Chapter 4

Sleep

JOAN L. F. SHAVER
and
ELIZABETH C. GIBLIN
DEPARTMENT OF PHYSIOLOGICAL NURSING
UNIVERSITY OF WASHINGTON

CONTENTS

Most people spend from one-quarter to one-third of their lives sleeping, yet investigations of sleep and function during sleep have been done to any extent only during the last 20 to 30 years. Sleep research is interdisciplinary, but to date little research has been done by nurses. However, increasing nurse involvement in sleep research is evident in the literature. The purpose of this chapter is to review

71

research related to sleep mainly reported in the nursing literature for its content, methodology, and the perspectives used to generate theory and to suggest potential research thrusts. Occasionally studies not part of nursing literature are mentioned because of their relevance to nursing considerations. Studies were accessed by a review of the *Cumulative Index to Nursing and Allied Health Literature* from 1971, Vol. *16*, to 1987, Vol. *32*, and a review of four nursing research journals: *Nursing Research, Research in Nursing and Health, Western Journal of Nursing Research*, and *Advances in Nursing Science*. All primary studies that could be accessed from various library holdings were included.

Sleep in humans has been measured by surveys of sleep experiences, sleep diaries or logs, observations of sleep behaviors, and somnography, which involves graphing of measurements obtained by use of the electroencephalograph (EEG), electrooculograph (EOG), and electromyograph (EMG). Self-report of sleep is difficult to obtain in a reliable form without missing data. The data are subject to bias in replies and are influenced by the motivation of subjects. Observational methods are difficult to use reliably and require extensive time commitment and vigilance of effort. However, from a nursing perspective, both are feasible methods of data collection. Somnography is presently the major method by which sleep patterns are quantified, but it is done most accurately in the laboratory, a practice that presents an artificial environment, which could in its own way influence sleep patterns. The method presently lacks feasibility for clinical or home assessment, but it does allow for finite assessment of sleep stages. Somnographic measurement is cumbersome technically and requires extensive expenditure of time and is therefore expensive.

In general, current interdisciplinary research into sleep has been addressed to the following aspects of sleep: (a) the neural regulation of sleep, using animals; (b) the effects of sleep deprivation and manipulation of environmental cues in humans or animals to determine the function of sleep, using mainly an experimental approach; (c) normal sleep and physiological function during sleep in healthy individuals across the age span, from an epidemiological perspective; (d) sleep patterns associated with various disease and illness states or with altered physiological functioning such as pregnancy; (e) sleep disorders such as sleep apnea, primary insomnia, and narcolepsy; (f) sleep as affected by environmental factors, such as rotating shifts or traveling across time zones; and (g) sleep in nonhome environments, such as hospitals or nursing homes. The majority of sleep research reported in the nursing literature relates to normal sleep in healthy individuals or sleep in the nonhome environment.

Much sleep research has been targeted at generating normative data about sleep patterns or determining the prevalence of sleep problems in various age groups, using both subjective and objective methodology. Such knowledge is fundamental to developing a basis for diagnosing abnormalities. In the search for generalizable information about sleep patterns, investigators have shown that wide variation exists among individuals. Therefore, much more research is needed to determine the range of sleep patterns in individuals and the circumstances influencing sleep.

Physiological stability–instability patterning or change during sleep also has been studied and is of interest in predicting sleep stages that might be detrimental for vulnerable populations, particularly those individuals who are ill. Sleep patterns occurring in states of altered health have been investigated mainly by clinicians in medicine.

SLEEP AS A BEHAVIOR

Sleep is a state of active, heterogeneous, neurophysiological functioning, synchronized with the light–dark cycle of the environment and characterized by cycling of the stages of sleep throughout the sleep period time. Essentially, human sleep is designated as nonrapid eye movement (NREM) sleep and rapid eye movement (REM) sleep according to the absence or presence of conjugal eye movements as monitored on an electrooculogram (EOG). During NREM sleep, electroencephalogram (EEG) waveforms increasingly become synchronized, slower in frequency, and of greater amplitude as deeper sleep ensues. The EEG waveforms are used to determine Stage 1, a transition stage from waking to sleeping; Stage 2, light sleep; and Stages 3 and 4, deep sleep, slow wave sleep (SWS), or delta sleep (Robinson, 1986). The difference between Stages 3 and 4 is in the proportion of delta waves per time period of measurement, with the proportion higher in Stage 4.

The skeletal muscle tension as monitored by electromyogram

(EMG) during deep sleep is less than during most waking circumstances, but only slightly so. Physiological indicators, for example, heart rate, ventilation rate, and blood pressure, during NREM sleep show general slowing compared to waking state but are fairly stable. In contrast, during REM sleep the EEG recording shows a rather desynchronized wave pattern similar to waking, but postural muscle tone disappears. Physiological indicators during REM sleep are much less stable and show more erratic changes than in NREM sleep (Robinson, 1986).

In general, the main variables of the sleep somnogram are: (a) latency to sleep onset (SOL), referring to the time taken to fall asleep; (b) latency to various stages; (c) the percent of time spent in each of the stages, including awake after sleep onset; and (d) the distribution of the sleep stages over the sleep period time (SPT).

Sleep stability is judged by the variables of: (a) sleep efficiency index, referring to the time spent sleeping per time spent in bed; (b) arousal index, referring to the number of sleep stage changes from deep sleep to awakening or to Stage 1 and lasting less than 10 seconds per hour; and (c) fragmentation index, referring to the number of stage changes to a lighter stage of sleep or to waking per hour.

Using subjective measurement, various sleep pattern variables also can be measured and include estimated sleep latency, intercurrent awake time, number of awakenings, and total time in bed. Aspects of sleep quality also can be assessed, such as satisfaction with sleep, soundness of sleep, quality of sleep, and feelings of being rested or clearheaded after the sleep period time.

INDIVIDUAL ADAPTATIONS: SLEEP DURING WELLNESS

Using somnography, much research has been done to determine normative sleep patterns (Williams, Karachan, & Hursch, 1974). Most of this work has not been done by nurse scientists except for a few studies related to sleep in infants (Edgil, Wood, & Smith, 1985; Friedemann & Emrich, 1978; Osterholm, Lindeke, & Amidon, 1983) and in the elderly (Hayter, 1983). Sleep is known to change with age, and a brief overview of sleep across age groups is included as background for the reviewed studies.

Young Adults

In usually less than 10 minutes, the young adult normally enters Stage 1 NREM sleep upon retiring, next descends into Stage 2, then into deep sleep (Stages 3 and 4), and enters REM sleep to complete one sleep cycle in about 90 minutes. This pattern repeats itself four to five times over the night. Deep sleep is proportionally greater early in the sleep period, and more and longer REM periods occur toward morning for night sleepers. The total sleep time for most young adults (20 to 35 years of age) is between 6 and 9 hours (Winegard & Berkman, 1983).

Infants and Children

Full-term newborns exhibit variable amounts of sleep interruptions, presumably because of hunger, environmental conditioning, or insufficient development of diurnal periodicity (Ferber, 1985). Somnographs show that infants at birth have even distribution of REM (active sleep) and NREM (quiet) periods, more time spent in REM sleep (50%) than adults (20%) per 24 hours, routine REM onset, and a shorter REM–NREM sleep cycle (50 to 60 minutes) than adults (60 to 90 minutes). Average total sleep time per 24 hours for normal-term babies has been reported as 13 to 16 hours (Anders, 1981; Barnard, 1985; Parmalee & Stern, 1972). By the second year of life, a reduction in the proportion of REM sleep and a progressive shift in REM sleep to the latter third of the night is apparent.

Interestingly, sleeplessness in the form of bedtime difficulties or nighttime awakenings is said to be the most common sleep problem of infancy and the toddler years (Ferber, 1985). Although somnographic data provide evidence that after 6 months of age sleep as a diurnal phenomenon is established, survey data showed that 25% of children 6 to 12 months still were waking up regularly. Of children 14 to 27 months of age, 23% to 44% were found to be waking up (Ferber, 1985).

Between the ages of 6 and 12 years, sleep duration in children decreases from a mean of 9 to 7.5 hours, Stage 4 declines from about 18% to 14% with increased Stage 2 sleep, and REM sleep remains relatively constant (Coble, Kupfer, Taska, & Kane, 1984). A progressive increase in the proportion of Stage 4 sleep from preadolescence to late adolescence appears (see Anders, 1981, for review), but decreases as sexual maturity is reached. Clinically, teenagers are said to have increased daytime sleepiness and possibly sleep deprivation, but this observation remains controversial.

In the nursing literature, three studies were found in which investigators surveyed sleep in healthy children at home. In an early study of sleep at home in normal infants, investigators examined sleep–wake patterns in conjunction with mothers' perceptions of ideal sleep patterns for their children (Friedemann & Emrich, 1978). No demographic or sampling information was provided, but mothers were approached in the hospital. An Infant Wake Schedule, Infant Activity Scale, and interview about behaviors were developed by the authors; as well, the Zuckerman Multiple Affect Adjective Checklist (Zuckerman, 1960) was used to measure maternal anxiety. When infants were 2 weeks of age, mothers wished that infants would sleep more ($M = 11.05$ hours) than they did ($M = 8.01$ hours). The discrepancy between actual and desired awake time declined but was still present at 12 weeks. Of the 38 infant–mother pairs in the sample, age at which infants began to sleep through the night ranged from 0 to 11 weeks, with a mean of 5.4 weeks. Maternal anxiety scores on a checklist instrument did not correlate with infant's age of initiating all-night sleep, nor did other factors related to pregnancy, labor, delivery, postpartum, or parenting.

In the second study, investigators used data from a mailed questionnaire on infant sleep problems and 5-day sleep records received from 80 families and showed that the prevalence of sleep disturbances in children 6 to 12 months was 44% ($N = 35$) (Osterholm et al., 1983). Subgroups of 35 sleep-disturbed infants and 45 infants who did not awaken at night were compared on selected characteristics. Breastfed babies and children who slept in their parents' rooms had a higher incidence of night awakenings. In this study, reliability and validity of the instruments were not reported. The sample was not selected randomly, and although demographic characteristics were not reported, the sample likely was fairly homogeneous. Precisely which variables were used for statistical analyses was unspecified. The findings did corroborate the rather high prevalence of sleep stability disturbances in this age group already reported in the literature (Ferber, 1985).

In the third study Edgil et al. (1985) surveyed 40 mother–child pairs in which the children were 9 to 48 months old. Twenty of the mothers reported at a private-practice pediatric visit that they were "satisfied" with their children's sleep, and the remainder reported being "not satisfied" with their children's sleep. Histories and 7-day sleep behavior records were completed by the mothers. A statistically significant difference (statistic not specified) in average total sleep time was found between the groups (no sleep problems, M = 10.6 hours and sleep problems, M = 7.5 hours). The majority of mothers (70%) reported that sleep problems of their children caused "little" to "moderate" disruption in family functioning. This study was described as using a convenience sample of middle-class families, although demographics were unspecified. Neither information about prevalence of sleep problems nor details about possible mechanisms were discernible in this study.

Environmental factors of various types may influence sleeping behaviors at home. It has been determined that children normally awaken during the night. One view is that children then must fall asleep several times during the night. If the sleep initiation is associated with circumstances such as being held, rocked, nursed, or suckled, then the absence of such factors at other nighttime awakenings may interfere with ease of falling back to sleep (Ferber, 1985). Caregiver behavior modification to promote sleep in children could be investigated as a nursing intervention.

A factor that might influence the sleeping habits of children and should interest nurses is feeding schedule, particularly nighttime feeding schedules. One recent study, not reported by nurses, produced evidence that the weaning status of infants influenced sleep patterns (Elias, Nicholson, Bora, & Johnston, 1986). Families were visited eight times over 2 years when infants were 2, 4, 7, 10, 13, 16, 20, and 24 months of age; parents were interviewed and a 24-hour feeding–sleep record collected (N = 32). Infants breastfed into their second year had short sleep periods with frequent awakenings when compared to those who were weaned at a median age of 12.75 months. Total sleep in 24 hours was less than that of weaned infants. This pattern was most obvious in infants who both were nursed and shared a bed with their mothers.

It has been shown previously that breastfed babies wake more (Ferber, 1985; Osterholm et al., 1983). One might question whether the rather continuous feeding that occurs with nursing throughout the night disrupts the circadian rhythms associated with episodic eating confined to the daytime, the more adult pattern of feeding for human beings. Although sleeping behaviors seem to be affected by feeding behaviors, little work has been done to clarify the effects on health status. Do the interpersonal and nutritive aspects of frequent feedings that seemingly interrupt the length of sleep periods provide benefit to the developing individual beyond any benefit that would be derived from longer sleep periods?

Aged Adults

Older individuals have been found to have an impaired capacity to maintain sleep. Findings in somnographic studies showed that wake time after sleep onset, number of nocturnal awakenings, duration of awakenings, and final awake time were all increased in older age groups (Bixler, Kales, Jacoby, Solkatos, & Vela-Bueno, 1984; Feinberg, 1974; Webb & Campbell, 1980, Williams et al., 1974). Older adults have more difficulty falling back to sleep than do younger sleepers. Sleep latency has been reported to be lengthened (Hayashi & Endo, 1982) or to show no change (Bixler et al., 1984). Stage 4 deep sleep declines rapidly with age; there is an increase in Stage 1 and in the number of shifts to Stage 1. A decline in the amount of REM sleep occurs, and its distribution becomes more uniform during the night (Hayashi & Endo, 1982).

While somnography to generate normative information has not been reported in the nursing literature, one study (Hayter, 1983) was found in nursing in which findings corroborated some of these same sleep changes with data collected by survey questionnaire. Mailed questionnaires and sleep diaries were kept by 212 healthy, community-based subjects aged 65 to 93 years. A significant increase in time in bed, total sleep time when naps were counted, number and amount of naps, and number and amount of wake time after sleep onset was apparent after age 75 when age groups were compared by chi-square analysis. These data support the notions that more time is spent in rest and sleep in old age; that sleep is more fragmented; and that it returns to a distribution that is more even throughout the 24 hours, much like it starts out in infancy. Because sleep distribution is a function of social scheduling, and this factor often is less structured in old age, it remains to be determined how the social environment contributes to sleep patterning in older adults.

Descriptive studies of normative sleep patterns in individuals across the life span done by investigators from many disciplines have served to provide some generalizable aspects of sleep, but mainly they have indicated wide variations among individuals. Much more work is needed in categorizing subtypes of responders and determining the factors that predict sleep patterns or sleep quality. Data from existing nursing studies have suggested that the sleep stability of infants and older adults may be a problem and that aspects of the social environment might affect sleep behaviors. No theoretical framework for explaining diminished sleep stability has been explicated or tested.

ENVIRONMENTS: SLEEP IN INSTITUTIONS

Much of nursing practice involves manipulating the environment in order to reduce challenges or provide modified inputs to individuals, families, or groups that need to heal themselves or advance their self-care practices. Because much nursing is done in institutions, particularly hospitals, research into behaviors exhibited in hospitals commonly is considered relevant to nursing practice. Several studies have been done on sleep of infants and children in hospitals, aged individuals in institutions, and ill persons in hospitals, particularly critical care environments.

Hospitalized Infants and Children

Two nursing studies were found in which sleep patterns of healthy newborns were investigated in relation to the influence of various hospital environmental factors. A comparative study was conducted of 20 healthy preterm infants placed in a nursery having nighttime light intensity and noise reduction and 21 healthy preterm infants placed in the usual nursery situation of constant light and noise. The results showed that infants in the reduced noise and light conditions slept for longer periods of time, took less time feeding, and gained more weight than the others (Mann, Hasddow, Stokes, Goodley, & Rutter, 1986). Differences between the groups were not significant statistically at discharge but were significant at the expected date of delivery (EDD), at EDD plus 6 weeks, and at EDD plus 12 weeks. Data collection for this study was done by many people, including nurses and mothers; no reliability checks of the sleep observations were done, and the observers presumably were not blind to the test conditions. However, the results are of potential interest to a framework of person–environment fit, problems of the hospital environment, and healthy behavior development.

In another study, Keefe (1987) made comparisons of the behavior of 11 normal newborns who roomed-in with their mothers at night with 10 who were cared for in the nursery. Measurement of behavior involved use of an infant state bassinet monitor with validity checked by observer scoring. Data were scored manually, with interrater reliability reported as 91.1%. The nursery environment was shown to have greater light and sound levels than the mothers' rooms. Infants in the mothers' rooms had significantly more quiet sleep, more total sleep, less indeterminate sleep, and less crying.

Considering more vulnerable populations of infants, preterm infants show diminished behavioral state integration. Sleep–wake cycling patterns have been used to represent the stability of the central nervous system in controlling physiological function relative to sensory input (Barnard, 1973), and an increase in indeterminate sleep is believed to indicate poor state integration. The variables used to determine sleep state were not concordant in all studies, but undifferentiated or indeterminate sleep state that is neither active nor quiet sleep was evident a larger proportion of the time in preterm babies than in term infants (Anders, 1981). The proportion of active sleep was elevated, and quiet sleep was reduced compared to full-term infant sleep.

Preterm infants as a group of individuals vulnerable to deteriorating health status have been studied by Barnard (1973). Rather than surveying environmental factors potentially associated with sleep disruption or selecting environments that differed in potential sleep disruption levels, manipulation of the environment to promote positive sleep pattern adaptations formed the basis for this research. Regulation of auditory (heartbeat sounds) and kinesthetic (timed rocking bed) stimulation for infants during weeks 33 and 34 of gestation were tested for their effects on sleep–wake behaviors, general maturation, and weight gain. A gain in the proportion of quiet sleep and a reduction in active sleep were observed in the test group, whereas the comparison group did the opposite. This result was accompanied by a larger weight gain and more neurological development in the test group. The findings for the groups were not different statistically; however, the test group started at a lower mean gestational age at the beginning of the study, so they achieved greater gains to stay comparable with the comparison group.

These studies carry implications that factors of the environment, including physical ones, affect sleep behaviors of infants and young children. Furthermore, they provide evidence that sleep quality influences health status, at least in the maturing individual. Therefore, manipulation of the environment to influence sleep for therapeutic health status outcomes warrants further study.

Findings of another study of sleep in high-risk, ill, or preterm infants documented the sleep disruption associated with hospitalization. Duxbury, Broz, and Wachdorf (1984) looked at caregiver disruptions as related to sleep in high-risk infants cared for in a neonatal intensive care unit. Forty-eight infants selected by random, representative methods were observed on 74 occasions in 3-hour blocks and over evenly distributed times of the day and days of the week. The average number of disruptions for 222 infant hours of observation was 2.13 times per hour, with the average hourly duration being 14 minutes. Caregiving procedures related to activities of daily living and comfort accounted for 28%, observation and monitoring for 38%, and treatments for 34% of the disruptions. Nurses were the most frequent disruptors, and disruptions occurred evenly over the hours of the day. Mean sleep time (118.3 ± 34.7 minutes), awakenings (3.55 ± 2.2 times), and lapse time between disturbances (30.2 ± 24.3 minutes) were reported for an average 3-hour block. Total sleep time was not related to severity of illness, although infants who were most critically ill were disrupted more often and for longer periods.

Three studies of sleep in older children in hospitals were found in the nursing literature. One by Hagemann (1981a) was an observational study of sleep in a convenience sample of 34 children, aged 3 to 8 years, who were admitted for elective surgery or with a medical condition requiring diagnostic testing. Subjects were observed for approximately 15 to 30 seconds every 5 minutes from 8:00 P.M. to 8:30 A.M. the following day. Results showed that the total duration of sleep between 8:00 P.M. and 8:30 A.M. ranged in duration from 4 to 10.5 hours ($M = 7.9$ hours). The average amount of sleep obtained represented a loss of one-fifth to one-quarter of usual sleep time. Sleep onset ranged from 8:00 P.M. to 1:45 A.M. Sleep termination occurred between 4:30 A.M. and 8:30 A.M. Sleep disruptions ($M = 3.5$ disruptions per child) were analyzed as being of an internal nature, such as hunger, or an external nature, such as noise (Hagemann, 1981b). The range of sleep disruptions was none to 17. Most disruptions were caused by external factors.

Findings in an earlier observational study of sleep during children's naptimes in the hospital for 24 3- to 5-year-olds over 4 to 6 days showed that the mean duration of time for napping was 76 minutes, with a range of 54 to 94 minutes (Beardslee, 1976). Sleep duration was 41 minutes on average. Sleep disruptions, defined as instances when children had fallen asleep, were aroused, and remained awake for the remainder of scheduled naptimes, were observed 40% of the time. Generally arousals were caused by a noisy environment and disruption by the staff. Sampling procedures and criteria for judging sleep were not explicated, and only descriptive analysis was done for this study.

The third study involved testing a parent-voice, tape-recorded story to influence sleep onset latency in hospitalized children 3 to 8 years old (White, Wear, & Stephenson, 1983). Observations were done for three consecutive nights on a convenience sample of 18 children. Although no statistically significant differences between the "story" and "no story" groups were seen, the test group did fall asleep slightly faster. A rather elaborate system of recording falling-asleep behaviors was used and categories of falling-asleep behaviors generated. Whereas this study was meant to test a therapy to promote sleep, a major portion of the study report instead was used to describe the development of sleep behavior coding.

Institutionalized Elderly

Five studies in the nursing literature were related to the sleep of institutionalized older persons. One observational study on a skilled care unit with a convenience sample of three males and eight females 60 to 97 years old gave evidence that nocturnal sleep behaviors, not surprisingly, were variable among individuals; some had severely disrupted sleep (Gress, Bahr, & Hassanein, 1981). Observations were made hourly by two nurse researchers. No attempt was made to look at subtypes of responders, obviously difficult with such a small sample. The criteria for determining sleep were unspecified, as was the length of the observation period. No reliability and validity of measurement were mentioned. Results did not suggest any factors involved in the observed disrupted sleep.

Bahr and Gress (1985) reported another study of 12 individuals (three male and nine female) ranging in age from 67 to 93 years. Observation of subjects for 30 seconds every 30 minutes was done, and interrater reliability was reported as 98%. The main purposes were to determine the 24-hour sleep–wakefulness pattern and any differences or variations occurring over 72 hours. The data description was minimal, but according to graphed data, the majority of sleep took place during the nighttime hours. The individual variation was substantial, and few generalizations were possible with the small sample size.

Johnson (1985) reported a study of a convenience sample of 75 ambulatory older subjects in a long-term care facility. Self-report of nocturnal behaviors, sleep variables, and daytime behaviors were described, and the effect of selected sleeping medications on these variables determined. The results were not reported according to statistical significance, making interpretation of the data uncertain. However, regardless of drug intake, subjects reported prolonged sleep onset latencies and light to medium sleep. Females tended to have a higher incidence of subjective sleep complaints than males; no relationship of sleep problems to age was evident, and sleep patterns were more disturbed in subjects taking benzodiazepines. Daytime activities were reported to be little affected by sleep medications.

A fourth study was done using an interview questionnaire on current as well as preadmission sleep in 102 elderly patients in three long-term-care facilities (Clapin-French, 1986). Based only on frequency statistics, results showed that patients reported napping more after admission than before, having more nocturnal interruptions in sleep (especially due to elimination and the proximity of other people), and going to bed earlier than at home. Seventy-one percent of the patients were receiving sleep medications.

These studies provided supporting evidence that institutionalization in long-term-care facilities has disrupted sleep patterns. However, little information was reported from these studies on diagnostic categories of sleep, factors associated with sleep problems, or the effects of sleep patterns on psychological or physiological functioning.

In the previous studies, comparison of institutional sleep with preadmission sleep was not done or done only by recall. However, Pacini and Fitzpatrick (1982) reported on a cross-sectional comparison study of 38 older individuals aged 60 to 82 years, half of whom were hospitalized in an acute-care facility and half not. Interestingly, results showed that both groups reported comparable amounts of sleep per 24 hours, but the pattern of obtaining the sleep differed. Total sleep time did not differ significantly between groups, but nocturnal sleep time and other sleep time did. Hospitalized patients went to bed and awakened earlier; but sleep latency, nocturnal arousals, and soundness of sleep did not differ from people at home. Variables such as self-rated health status, state of mind, and fatigue (measurement unspecified) differed between the groups. When these variables were controlled for by analysis of covariance, they appeared to influence sleep beyond the impact of the hospital environment.

In sum, of these five studies, two (Bahr & Gress, 1985; Gress et al., 1981) were done using observations by nurse researchers. In the remainder, investigators used self-report and questionnaires. Two studies (Johnson, 1985; Pacini & Fitzpatrick, 1982) were performed using a self-report sleep pattern questionnaire derived by Baekeland and Hoy (1971), whereas in the investigation by Clapin-French (1986), new instruments were generated. Interestingly, none of the authors mentioned that the subjects, some of whom were advanced in age, had difficulty completing the instruments accurately.

The issue of self-report sleep measurement remains an important one and has been addressed by one team of nurse scientists. A visual analogue instrument to measure perceived sleep quality has been derived and tested by Snyder-Halpern and Verran (1987). It contains a sleep disturbance factor with items related to sleep latency, midsleep awakenings, soundness of sleep, and movement during sleep and an effectiveness factor with items related to rested feelings upon awakening, subjective quality of sleep, and total sleep period. The instrument has been found to have adequate reliability (theta = .82) and scale validity, using factor analysis and tests of convergent construct validity by correlating items with corresponding items on the St. Mary's Hospital Sleep Questionnaire (Ellis et al., 1981). Further development of this instrument is planned. If it continues to exhibit sound psychometric properties, it has much promise for providing some consistency to sleep self-report data and for generating cumulative nursing knowledge.

Critical Care Environments

Findings in several studies in the nursing literature have documented that sleep deprivation occurs in intensive care environments because of patients not being given time to sleep. Sleep deprivation has been of interest as a contributing factor to postoperative psychosis. An early study by McFadden and Giblin (1971) was done to determine whether sleep deprivation existed following open-heart surgery. Results of sleep observations in four patients showed that there were hardly any periods of time in which patients received at least 60 minutes of uninterrupted time for rest over six postoperative days. Three of four patients experienced unusual cognitive-behavioral changes. In similar studies of four postcardiotomy patients each, Walker (1972) and Woods (1972) showed that none of the subjects obtained uninterrupted time for complete sleep cycles, with the majority of interruptions being attributed to the nurses. Woods (1972) reported that two of four subjects had unusual behavioral manifestations. These studies were nonrepresentative, small sample studies that have served to attract attention to the environmentally imposed sleep deprivation in critical care. In a study in a respiratory intensive care unit, Hilton (1976) observed, using EEG recordings, that patients experienced significant reductions in REM and SWS sleep time.

Helton, Gordon, and Nunnery (1980) used a larger sample size ($N = 62$) and more systematic measurement of mental status. Altered mental state was scored according to severity of mental symptoms, although consistent raters apparently were not used, nor were any inter-rater reliability checks reported. Potential sleep cycles were considered present when at least 75 minutes were available for sleep without interruptions, as documented on an interruption checklist completed by the intensive care unit staff or the researchers. Cumulative sleep deprivation was calculated. Subjects were divided into categories of not deprived, moderately deprived (50% loss of potential sleep), and severely sleep-deprived (greater than 50% loss of potential sleep). On day 3 in the ICU, 19 out of 55 patients were moderately or severely sleep-deprived. This result documented a level of sleep deprivation that was less than in the previously mentioned studies, perhaps because of the larger sample size, less precise measurements, or the development of awareness of sleep deprivation in intensive care nurses. Alternately, data collection methods may have sensitized the staff nurses to the amount of sleep deprivation being incurred, resulting in altered usual practices.

Subjects who were deprived of sleep were significantly (Fischer's exact correlation) more likely to exhibit symptoms of altered mental status than those who were not sleep-deprived (Helton et al., 1980). However, only 11% of the total sample and one-third of those severely sleep-deprived showed some mental status changes on the third postoperative day. This finding is less than some investigators have reported, but factors such as selection and exclusion criteria or lack of sensitivity of the mental status assessment, as pointed out by the authors, might have influenced prevalence.

Sleep deprivation in critical care patients often has been attributed to noise (Hilton, 1976). A laboratory study of sleep in healthy subjects exposed to noise, taped from an actual ICU setting, showed that exposure to ICU noise during sleep was associated with increased cardiac rates and self-reported poor sleep when compared to "quiet" nights of sleep (Snyder-Halpern, 1985). This study was performed with a small sample and had nonrandom application of the independent variable, and the investigator neglected to specify whether the subjects or coders were blind to the test conditions. However, it was one of the few studies to include investigation of the physiological effects of environmental noise during sleep. A laboratory study of similar type might be done while sleep is monitored polygraphically to determine corollary sleep pattern effects.

In sum, nursing research regarding sleep in infants, children, and adults who were hospitalized has provided evidence that physical environmental factors such as light and noise have a negative effect on sleep behaviors. As well, the delivery of nursing care or lack of environmental control of disruptions for sick infants, children, and adults leads to sleep deprivation. Little work has been done to determine the effects of disrupted sleep in these environments on health status or on the testing of environmental manipulation to promote sleep.

Findings in early studies with small samples have implied that little time for sleep is available to critically ill patients and that environmental factors such as noise, light, and caregiving activities interfere with sleep potential. Whether patients are deprived selectively of certain sleep stages is not certain, given that polygraphic studies are sparse. Sleep is believed to have restorative purposes, and sleep deprivation has been associated with reduced protein synthesis and immunosuppression (Palmblad, Petrini, Wasserman, & Akerstedt, 1979), suggesting that poor sleep might be associated with negative health status outcomes. No studies were found in which indicators such as incidence of infection, wound healing rates, other complications, or length of hospitalization in relation to sleep difficulties were measured. The effect of sleep deprivation on cognitive-emotional status still is not clear. Cumulative research through multiple studies using comparable methodologies is not available but is needed.

INDIVIDUAL ADAPTATIONS: SLEEP AND ILLNESS

Physiological or psychological function during sleep or the effect of sleep on physiological or psychological function in vulnerable individuals, such as those who are ill or diseased, has been studied, though not extensively. Because much nursing practice occurs in the context of major illness, knowledge of sleep accompanying major disease and illness states, although rarely investigated by nurse scientists, potentially is relevant to nursing science.

Cardiopulmonary Function

Cardiopulmonary diseases are major ailments in highly developed, Western cultures. Knowledge of the effects of sleep states on cardiopulmonary function could have clinical implications for a number of patients or clients cared for in the community or hospital.

Cardiovascular function is affected by sleep in healthy individuals. Blood pressure and heart rate fall during NREM sleep, with increased variability during REM sleep. Cardiac output falls in all stages of sleep. Sinus pauses occur in about 30% of subjects aged 40 to 79 years. Heart block and ventricular arrhythmias can occur in normal subjects during sleep, but no consistency between these and sleep state has been demonstrated (Gillis, 1985). The association of premature ventricular contractions (PVCs) with sleep is unclear. Some coronary care patients have shown more PVCs during waking; some show more during REM, and some show more during NREM sleep. In some individuals, PVCs disappear during sleep (Gillis, 1985). Patients with sleep apnea syndrome or chronic obstructive lung disease have more frequent PVCs at night than during the day. Cyclical bradycardia followed by tachycardia occurs so consistently with apneic episodes that monitoring of heart function can serve as a screening diagnostic test for sleep apnea (Motta & Guilleminault, 1985). In general, no evidence exists that any sleep provokes life-threatening ventricular arrhythmias in the general population.

Sleep apnea (the cessation of breathing during sleep) is the focus for much research (Orr, 1983). Apneic episodes vary in duration and frequency and create variable risk of hypoxemia because of blood oxygen desaturation. The episodes may occur as central apneas associated with abnormal regulation of ventilatory effort by the brain, as an obstructive phenomenon because of inadequate control of the tissues of the pharynx, or as a mixture of the two problems. Common symptoms and signs are daytime sleepiness or fatigue, usually believed caused by a high number of arousals from sleep; hypersomnolence; snoring; arrhythmias; hypoxemia; systemic hypertension; right ventricular failure; and pulmonary hypertension. Long-range effects are pulmonary hypertension occurring in response to hypoxemia, which creates increased resistance to right heart pumping and the potential for right-sided heart failure. Treatments for moderate to severe manifestations are tracheostomy, reconstruction of the upper airway tissues, called a uvulopalatopharyngoplasty, or sometimes drug treatment in the form of medroxyprogesterone or protriptyline. Recent treatments include continuous positive airway pressure (CPAP) or continuous low-flow oxygen during sleep. For less severe cases, weight loss therapy and devices to prevent a back-lying position sometimes can be useful therapeutically.

Nursing studies of this condition are sparse. It is not a sleep disorder, but rather a sleep-related breathing disorder that can have dire consequences if not treated. Nursing research might include studies on the effect of this condition, particularly some of the medical therapies, on quality of life. Clinical observations are that CPAP is associated with poor compliance. Research related to health teaching, support, and behavioral modification for health maintenance and promotion would be warranted for nursing science. No such nursing studies were evident in the literature.

Cancer and Trauma

Isolated descriptive studies related to sleep and the illness categories of cancer, burns, and head injuries have been reported in the nursing literature. One recent study on sleep patterns of hospitalized cancer patients compared to patterns of noncancer patients ($N = 30$) was done using self-report measures of anxiety, depression, and sleep difficulties (Lamb, 1982). Although depression in the hospital was significantly greater than recalled depressive characteristics at home in the oncology patients, sleep problems were not significantly different between the groups. A trend for more sleep complaints in the oncology patients was seen, however. The author pointed to several possible factors, including lack of a sensitive instrument to measure sleep quality, as affecting the outcomes. It should be noted that measurement occurred within 24 hours of hospital admission and again "a few" days before discharge rather than at more frequent times.

In another singular study reported in the nursing literature, Dotson, Kibbee, and Eland (1986) reported on the assessment of night sleep in burn patients. Measurement included a preburn history of usual sleep period length and daily postburn self-assessments of sleep quality, satisfaction with sleep, and sleep period time. The average preburn sleep period time was reported as 8 hours per night, and the estimated postburn sleep period length at night over 20 days in 12 subjects was 6 hours per night; but this was not a statistically significant difference from at home preburn. Postburn sleep satisfaction was reduced compared to preburn recalled satisfaction, although statistical significance was not mentioned. These investigators had a small sample of 12 subjects, neglected to use correlational statistics for repeated measures when correlating over multiple days, and reported data in a table that was unclear as to which variables were correlated to each other, making it difficult to have confidence in the results. The measurement of sleep patterns in burn patients remains undocumented in the nursing literature.

Sleep patterns in head-injured patients have been studied minimally by nurse scientists. Parsons and Ver Beek (1982) reported on sleep patterns prior to injury and self-reported current sleep patterns in 75 subjects 3 months following minor head injury. Sleep interruptions per week and per night postinjury, time needed to function at peak efficiency upon awakening, and early morning awakenings all were increased. Sleep quality was decreased significantly. Although these findings imply altered sleep patterns after minor head injury, polysomnographic detailing is needed in order to guide therapy. The recall of preinjury sleep patterns is problematic. Therefore, it might be interesting to compare subjects experiencing a noncerebral injury to head injury patients for pre- and postinjury sleep alterations.

The postburn injury results by Dotson et al. (1986) also showed postinjury sleep deterioration, but these data were collected in the hospital. Sleep pattern assessment at home and longitudinal measurement in any injured patients would be of interest. Data obtained by intermittent sleep laboratory measurement as well as survey questionnaire would seem potentially lucrative for knowledge generation about sleep patterns in relation to illness and injury.

SUMMARY AND FUTURE RESEARCH DIRECTIONS

Nursing studies related to sleep are sparse in the literature. Some surveys have been done of people across the life span living in their own environments. Description of sleep in institutional environments primarily has been documentation of time for sleep or lack thereof and environmental factors that are presumable disruptors of sleep for patients. Such knowledge does have some direct implications for the delivery of nursing care services and for altering the environments in institutions.

Several topics were covered in the literature, but there were few studies within each topic, making it difficult to analyze cumulative knowledge. Most studies lacked a theoretical perspective, and few continuing studies have been done. Additionally, few investigators have addressed an evaluation of any therapies for sleep problems or have focused on using sleep as a therapeutic modality. Although it might be considered premature to suggest therapeutic interventions before adequate descriptive work is available, it can be argued that mechanisms sometimes are illuminated when therapeutic strategies are being tested.

The study of sleep by investigators in many disciplines has been done using a purely physiological perspective, with little consideration for psychosocial and sociocultural factors that might influence sleep pattern differences. Sleep might be considered a human response to real or potential health problems; but rather than focusing on sleep associated with individual medical diseases, it might be fruitful for nurses to study sleep during life transitions, grieving, and the stresses of acute and chronic illness. Although it seems natural to consider sleep as a response to or an indicator of altered health status and therefore to study the effect of health status on sleep, theoretically it also seems reasonable to study the effect of sleep patterns on health status.

Sleep also has been considered as a singular state of functioning, but sleep is manifested in a circadian pattern and needs to be considered from a perspective of person-environment fit. Little work in the nursing literature has been concerned with circadian factors and sleep-wake cycling except for two studies (Floyd, 1984; Leddy, 1977) that were reviewed elsewhere (Felton, 1987).

Studies about sleep patterns as a response to health problems, sleep as a health problem, sleep as a biopsychosocial phenomenon, and sleep as part of the sleep–wakefulness circadian pattern of human functioning barely have begun. Nursing research with theoretical bases that take these aspects into consideration is needed to contribute substantive knowledge to the science of caring related to health.

REFERENCES

Anders, T. T. (1981). The development of sleep patterns and sleep disturbances from infancy through adolescence. *Advances in Behavioral Pediatrics, 2,* 171–190.

Baekeland, F., & Hoy, P. (1971). Reported versus recorded sleep characteristics. *Archives of General Psychiatry, 24,* 548–551.

Bahr, R. T., & Gress, L. (1985). The 24-hour cycle: Rhythms of healthy sleep. *Journal of Gerontological Nursing, 11*(4), 14–17.

Barnard, K. (1973). The effect of stimulation on the sleep behavior of the premature infant. In M. V. Batey (Ed.), *Communicating nursing research* (Vol. 6) (pp. 12–23). Boulder, CO: Western Interstate Commission for Higher Education.

Barnard, K. (1985). Sleep behaviors of infants – Is it important? *NCAST National News, 1,* 1 & 4.

Beardslee, C. (1976). The sleep–wakefulness pattern of young hospitalized children during nap time. *Maternal–Child Nursing Journal, 5*, 15–24.

Bixler, E. O., Kales, A., Jacoby, J., Solkatos, C. R., & Vela-Bueno, A. (1984). Nocturnal sleep and wakefulness: Effects of age and sex in normal sleepers. *International Journal of Neuroscience, 23*, 33–42.

Clapin-French, E. (1986). Sleep patterns of aged persons in long-term care facilities. *Journal of Advanced Nursing, 11*, 57–66.

Coble, P. A., Kupfer, D. J., Taska, L. S., & Kane, J. (1984). EEG sleep of normal healthy children. Part 1: Findings using standard measurement methods. *Sleep, 7*, 289–303.

Dotson, C. H., Kibbee, E., & Eland, J. M. (1986). Perception of sleep following burn injury. *Journal of Burn Care Research, 7*, 105–108.

Duxbury, M. L., Broz, L. J., & Wachdorf, C. M. (1984). Caregiver disruptions and sleep of high-risk infants. *Heart & Lung, 13*, 141–147.

Edgil, A. E., Wood, K. L., & Smith, D. P. (1985). Sleep problems of older infants and preschool children. *Pediatric Nursing, 11*, 87–89.

Elias, M. F., Nicholson, N. A., Bora, C., & Johnston, J. (1986). Sleep/wake patterns of breastfed infants the first 2 years of life. *Pediatrics, 77*, 322–329.

Ellis, B., Johns, M. W., Lancaster, R., Raptopoulos, P., Angelopoulos, N., & Priest, R. (1981). The St. Mary's Hospital sleep questionnaire: A study of reliability. *Sleep, 4*, 93–97.

Feinberg, I. (1974). Changes in sleep cycle patterns with age. *Journal of Psychiatric Research, 10*, 283–306.

Felton, G. (1987). Human biologic rhythms. *Annual Review of Nursing Research, 5*, 45–77.

Ferber, R. (1985). Sleep, sleeplessness, and sleep disruptions in infants and young children. *Annals of Clinical Research, 17*, 227–234.

Floyd, J. A. (1984). Interaction between personal sleep–wake rhythms and psychiatric hospital rest–activity schedule. *Nursing Research, 33*, 255–259.

Friedemann, M. L., & Emrich, K. A. (1978). Emergence of infant sleep-awake patterns in the first three months after birth. *International Journal of Nursing Studies, 15*, 5–16.

Gillis, A. M. (1985). Cardiac arrhythmias during sleep. *Comprehensive Therapy, 11*(11), 66–71.

Gress, L. D., Bahr, R. T., & Hassanein, R. S. (1981). Nocturnal behavior of selected institutionalized adults. *Journal of Gerontological Nursing, 7*, 86–92.

Hagemann, V. (1981a). Night sleep of children in a hospital, Part I: Sleep duration. *Maternal–Child Nursing Journal, 10*, 1–14.

Hagemann, V. (1981b). Night sleep of children in a hospital, Part II: Sleep description. *Maternal–Child Nursing Journal, 10*, 127–141.

Hayashi, Y., & Endo, S. (1982). All-night sleep polygraphic recordings of healthy aged persons: REM and slow-wave sleep. *Sleep, 5*, 277–283.

Hayter, J. (1983). Sleep behaviors of older persons. *Nursing Research, 32*, 242–246.

Helton, M. C., Gordon, S. H., & Nunnery, S. L. (1980). The correlation between sleep deprivation and the intensive care unit syndrome. *Heart & Lung, 9*, 464–468.

Hilton, B. A. (1976). Quantity and quality of patients' sleep and sleep-disturbing factors in a respiratory intensive care unit. *Journal of Advanced Nursing, 1,* 453–468.

Johnson, J. V. (1985). Drug treatment for sleep disturbances: Does it really work? *Journal of Gerontological Nursing, 11*(8), 8–12.

Keefe, M. R. (1987). Comparison of neonatal nighttime sleep–wake patterns in nursery versus rooming-in environments. *Nursing Research, 36,* 140–144.

Lamb, M. A. (1982). The sleeping patterns of patients with malignant and non-malignant diseases. *Cancer Nursing, 5,* 389–396.

Leddy, S. (1977). Sleep and phase shifting of biological rhythms. *International Journal of Nursing Studies, 14,* 137–150.

Mann, N. P., Hasddow, R., Stokes, L., Goodley, S., & Rutter, N. (1986). Effect of night and day on preterm infants in a newborn nursery: Randomized trial. *British Medical Journal, 293,* 1265–1267.

McFadden, E. H., & Giblin, E. C. (1971). Sleep deprivation in patients having open-heart surgery. *Nursing Research, 20,* 249–254.

Motta, J., & Guilleminault, C. (1985). Cardiac function during sleep. *Annals of Clinical Research, 17,* 190–198.

Orr, W. C. (1983). Sleep-related breathing disorders—An update. *Chest, 84,* 475–480.

Osterholm, P., Lindeke, L. L., & Amidon, D. (1983). Sleep disturbances in infants aged 6–12 months. *Pediatric Nursing, 9,* 269–271.

Pacini, C. M., & Fitzpatrick, J. J. (1982). Sleep patterns of hospitalized and non-hospitalized aged individuals. *Journal of Gerontological Nursing, 8,* 327–332.

Palmblad, J., Petrini, B., Wasserman, J., & Akerstedt, T. (1979). Lymphocyte and granulocyte reactions during sleep deprivation. *Psychosomatic Medicine, 41,* 272–277.

Parmalee, A. H., & Stern, E. (1972). Development of states in infants. In C. D. Clements, D. P. Purpua, & E. F. Mayer (Eds.), *Sleep and the maturing nervous system* (pp. 199–228). New York: Academic Press.

Parsons, L. C., & Ver Beek, D. (1981). Sleep–awake patterns following cerebral concussion. *Nursing Research, 31,* 260–264.

Robinson, C. (1986). Impaired sleep. In V. K. Carrieri, A. M. Lindsey, & C. M. West (Eds.), *Pathophysiological phenomena in nursing* (pp. 390–417). Philadelphia: Saunders.

Snyder-Halpern, R. (1985). The effect of critical care unit noise on patient sleep cycles. *Critical Care Quarterly, 7*(4), 41–51.

Snyder-Halpern, R., & Verran, J. A. (1987). Instrumentation to describe subjective sleep characteristics in healthy subjects. *Research in Nursing and Health, 10,* 155–163.

Walker, B. B. (1972). The post-surgery heart patient: Amount of uninterrupted time for sleep and rest during the first, second and third postoperative days in a teaching hospital. *Nursing Research, 21,* 164–169.

Webb, W. B., & Campbell, S. S. (1980). Awakenings and the return to sleep in an older population. *Sleep, 3,* 41–46.

White, M. A., Wear, E., & Stephenson, G. (1983). A computer-compatible method for observing falling asleep behavior of hospitalized children. *Research in Nursing and Health, 6,* 191–198.

Williams, R. L., Karachan, I., & Hursch, C. (1974). *EEG of human sleep: Clinical applications.* New York: Wiley.

Winegard, D. L., & Berkman, L. F. (1983). Mortality risk associated with sleeping patterns among adults. *Sleep, 6,* 102–107.

Woods, N. F. (1972). Patterns of sleep in postcardiotomy patients. *Nursing Research, 21,* 347–352.

Zuckerman, M. (1960). The development of an affect adjective checklist for the measurement of anxiety. *Journal of Consultant Psychology, 24,* 457–462.

Chapter 5

Infection Control

ELAINE L. LARSON
SCHOOL OF NURSING
JOHNS HOPKINS UNIVERSITY

CONTENTS

Nosocomial infections, which are infections that develop as a result of events occurring in a health care setting, affect approximately 6% of patients in acute-care institutions, adding an average of at least 4 days to length of stay and causing or contributing to deaths of about 80,000 patients at a cost of at least $4 billion annually nationwide. Prevalence rates for infection in extended care and skilled nursing facilities are estimated to be between 10 and 40%, also adding significantly to the economic and social burden of infections in this country (Haley, 1986; Haley, Culver, White, Morgan, & Emori, 1985). It has been calculated that at least one-third of nosocomial infections can be prevented (Haley, Culver, White, Morgan, Emori, Munn, & Hooton, 1985). Risk reduction and prevention of infection clearly fit within the responsibilities and purview of nursing.

Helpful critiques by Drs. Arlene Butz and Denise Korniewicz, Johnson and Johnson/ SURGIKOS Postdoctoral Nursing Fellows in Infection Control, are gratefully acknowledged.

95

Florence Nightingale set the stage for a preeminent role for nursing in the practice of infection control. When she arrived at Scutari Hospital in the Crimea in 1855, the death rate among soldiers was 42%, primarily as a result of infectious diseases such as cholera, typhoid, typhus, and Crimean fevers. Within 4 months, the death rate was reduced to 2% as a result of Nightingale's hygienic and administrative reforms (Cohen, 1984). After her time in the Crimea, Nightingale continued her efforts for sanitary reform in the British military, schools, public health agencies, and hospitals.

Despite her influence in improving the public health and reducing infections, Nightingale rejected the germ theory and the idea of personal contagion, referring to transmission of diseases from person to person (Rosenberg, 1979). In *Notes on Hospitals* (1863) she attributed nosocomial infections to poor architectural design, overcrowding, inadequate fresh air and light, and general lack of cleanliness. The belief that contagion was associated with "miasmas" in the air was shared by many of her contemporary medical colleagues. Even though Nightingale had inadequate knowledge of the infectious process, she did the right things to prevent the spread of contagious diseases. Her ideas were the origin for "fever nursing," which consisted of barrier and sanitary practices adopted by schools of nursing and hospitals in the United States by the turn of the century.

The first formal, systematic efforts within nursing to use an empirical approach to investigate practices related to infection control were in the early 1970s with the formation of a specialty organization, The Association for Practitioners in Infection Control (APIC). This organization now has approximately 7,000 members, 85% of whom are registered nurses. In the early 1980s, two interdisciplinary journals focused specifically on infection control were founded, *The American Journal of Infection Control* and *Infection Control*. The bulk of nursing and interdisciplinary research in this field has been published in one of these journals. This chapter contains a review of nursing research published between June 1981 and June 1987 in nursing and infection control literature.

METHODS OF REVIEW

Three sources of published nursing research were used: *Index Medicus, Cumulative Index of Nursing and Allied Health Literature,* and the two infection control journals. The titles varied slightly because of change in subject headings over time.

For the purpose of this chapter, nursing research was defined as research related to infection control in which the principal author was a professional nurse *and* which met the three criteria proposed by Diers (1979) for nursing research: The study had the potential for improving patient care, for contributing to theory development and the body of scientific nursing knowledge, and it involved a phenomenon to which nurses have access and over which they have control. The scientific merit of the studies was judged according to criteria described by Cooper (1982) and Duffy (1985). Only those studies that met minimum standards for adequate research designs were included in this review.

A total of 86 research reports that met the defined criteria for nursing research and scientific merit were found in 16 different journals. In addition, another 92 studies were found in which one or more coauthors was a nurse. These were categorized under four major headings: epidemiologic studies; methods of infection control practice; program evaluations; and infection control in clinical nursing practice.

Nursing research categorized as epidemiologic studies (30.2% of the total research), methods of infection control practice (20.9%) and program evaluation (8.1%) are not discussed in this review. Studies directly related to infection control in clinical nursing practice were categorized into two general areas. Those related to barrier techniques (26 studies, 30.2%) included studies of isolation precautions, visitors, attire, and handwashing and aseptic technique. Studies addressed to the infection control implications of specific patient care practices (9 studies, 10.5%) dealt primarily with enteral and parenteral therapy and respiratory care. For this chapter, these 35 nursing research studies were reviewed.

INFECTION CONTROL IN CLINICAL NURSING PRACTICE

Barrier Techniques

Isolation Precautions. Isolation precautions have assumed a major role in most hospital infection control programs, and yet research to evaluate efficacy of these practices is sorely lacking. In 1985, Jackson and Lynch conducted a historical review of the origins and evolution of such practices as reflected in the *American Journal of Nursing* from 1900 to 1984. They found that isolation practices originated primarily from two sources: public health measures to curtail the spread of communicable diseases in the community (i.e., quarantine), and an adaptation of operating room practices on patient care units. The authors elucidated two major controversies: (a) an ongoing debate about the relative importance of air and the inanimate environment compared to person-to-person and direct contact as major modes of transmission of infectious agents, and (b) an ongoing debate between those who proposed isolation only for individuals known to harbor infectious organisms and those who proposed that contact with body substances from any individual should be considered as potentially infectious and handled with precautions.

One group of investigators (Larson, Hargiss, & Dyk, 1985) attempted to examine the influence of physical facilities on risk of infection by reviewing trends in infection in a neonatal intensive care unit over a period of months when an architectural change resulted in a threefold increase in space per infant. There were no significant differences either in rates of nosocomial infection or in colonization of babies with *Staphylococcus aureus* over the 52 months studied. However, there was a marked decrease in clusters of cross-infections occurring in the new unit, indicating that transmission between infants might have been reduced. Although other changes over time that could have accounted for differences in infection rates could not be ruled out completely, there were no differences in such factors as severity of illness, length of stay, number of infants intubated, and other parameters to describe the patient population, nor were there major staffing or policy and procedure changes during the study period. Results of this study indicated that although architectural design might modify the risk of epidemic spread of infections, it had little relationship to the overall rates, because most nosocomial infections did not occur in outbreaks but rather at lower endemic rates.

Other nursing research related to barrier techniques has been concerned with compliance and acceptability of isolation policies. Gilmore, Montgomerie, and Graham (1986) implemented a procedure-oriented, simplified isolation system and conducted a survey to evaluate staff acceptance of the system. The majority of the 66% of responding staff members judged the system to be an improvement, but the authors did not attempt to assess compliance with the system. They did, however, attempt to measure effectiveness of the system with regard to reducing cross-infections. They noted a 17% nonsignificant reduction in cross-infections with an index organism in conjunction with the new isolation system.

Larson (1983) conducted an observational study to determine the extent of compliance of patient care staff with isolation precautions. In 372 observations of all patients on isolation precautions during a 33-day time period, the majority of procedures were followed (type and duration of isolation, disposal of contaminated equipment). A very disturbing finding, however, was that physical contact with patients known to be infected was followed by staff handwashing only less than half of the time. Insufficient and/or inadequate handwashing has been confirmed by a number of medical and nursing investigators (Albert & Condie, 1981; Larson, 1985; Preston, Larson, & Stamm, 1981) and thus appears to be a major clinical problem.

Since the onset of the epidemic of acquired immunodeficiency syndrome (AIDS) in the early 1980s, increased attention has been focused on isolation techniques, not just as a measure to prevent infections between patients but to protect the health care practitioner as well. Nevertheless, as of January 1987, no articles were found in the nursing literature that were focused on the issue of efficacy of various levels of barrier techniques (e.g., gloves alone; gloves and eye coverings; gloves, masks, and gowns) in reducing cross-infections for AIDS or any other disease. Indeed, there is a paucity in the nursing research literature in general regarding nursing issues related to infection with the human immunodeficiency virus. From 1983 through June 1987, not a single research-based article on this subject was found in the English-language nursing literature (Larson, 1988). Infection control and other issues related to AIDS must be a major nursing research priority during the next decade and has been identified as such by the National Center for Nursing Research (National Institutes of Health, 1987). In addition, the practice of specific types of isolation techniques is not supported by a research base and warrants nursing investigation. Such investigation is of particular importance because of the trend toward universal precautions or body substance isolation based on recommendations from the Centers for Disease Control (*Federal Register,* 1987). Although the concept of body substance isolation has been developed and proposed primarily by nurses, no research has been reported that demonstrates its efficacy (Lynch, Jackson, Cummings, & Stamm, 1987).

Visitors.   In two studies, researchers have assessed the effect of sibling visitation and contact on bacterial colonization in neonates.

The first (Wranesh, 1982) was a retrospective chart review of infants born within a 1-month time period. The study group was comprised of infants exposed to sibling visitation in a rooming-in situation; controls were infants on the same unit who had not received sibling visits. The outcome variable was results of infant nasal and umbilical cultures obtained at hospital discharge. Although no significant differences were found between the two groups in types of organisms isolated, the sample size of 20 per group was very small, and many extraneous variables were not addressed (e.g., birth order, infections of mothers, whether infants were colonized in the delivery room).

In a follow-up study (Kowba & Schwirian, 1985), 44 newborns were studied prospectively. In Phase I, 23 infants were assigned with a block design to receive sibling visits in a visitation room; for the 21 control infants, siblings only viewed them through the nursery window. In Phase II, 66 additional infants (33 experimental and 33 control) were studied in a protocol modified to account for additional potentially confounding variables (e.g., exposure of control infants to sibling organisms carried by parents). A further design improvement over the first study was that infants were cultured immediately upon admission to the unit as well as at hospital discharge. Again, no significant differences in colonization rates for staphylococci or streptococci were noted between groups. Despite design flaws in the first study, the combined sample size of these two studies (150 babies) and the consistent results lend credibility to the conclusion that, given adequate screening protocols, it is safe to allow sibling visitation to neonates. Because of immature immune status, neonates are at higher risk of infection than older children. Thus, results of these studies might be generalized to older children with normal immune function as well.

A third study was conducted to evaluate the effect on infection rates of having parents assist with infant care in a special-care baby unit (Boxall, Orme, & Cruickshank, 1982). For 2 years before and 3 years after shared care was initiated, data regarding mortality rates and antibiotic use were used as indicators of risk of infection. There were no differences in either of these variables before and after implementation of shared care. Unfortunately, only raw numbers were reported, and actual infection rates were not presented. Because the study occurred over a period of 5 years, other temporally related factors that might have influenced these variables could not be ruled out. Nevertheless, this study was addressed to an important practice issue for nurses and, if verified in more controlled trials, has important implications for care in neonatal units.

Attire.   In several recent nursing studies in the newborn nursery and the operating room, researchers evaluated the influence on infections of wearing protective attire. Roberts, Hammes, and Gundersen (1986) conducted a retrospective review of 243 patient medical records. There were no differences in infection rates among patients when three different combinations of attire were worn by delivery room staff. This study was flawed, however, by small sample size, lack of control over extraneous variables, and reliance on the chart to detect infections. Renaud (1983) reported a decrease in umbilical colonization of infants in a normal newborn nursery when gowning by visitors on the postpartum ward was discontinued. It was not clear, however, whether visitors to the nursery during the control phase wore covergowns or not. Additionally, the comparison groups were not concurrent.

In a study with a similar objective, Campbell (1987) monitored infection and colonization rates of 100 infants. In the control group (*n* = 50 babies), family members wore covergowns in the nursery and postpartum ward; in the experimental group, no covergowns were worn. Again, there were no significant differences between the groups of infants with regard to umbilical colonization or infection at 2 weeks of age. Although the independent and dependent variables were well defined, the actual data regarding colonization and infection rates were not included in the paper. It is, therefore, not possible to make a determination about the statistical power of the study. Additionally, infants were not assigned randomly to study groups, and the control group was nonconcurrent.

Hunter and Williams (1985) evaluated the effect of eliminating mask-wearing in the labor room. There were 239 deliveries in the study group in which no masks were worn, and 259 in the control group in which masks were worn. Reductions in infection rates were found in both groups during the study, but greater reductions were reported in the no-mask group. Although each of the described studies has serious design limitations, the results are very consistent with findings from larger and better-controlled trials in medical literature (Donowitz, 1986; Forfar & McCabe, 1958). Taken together, one can conclude that universal use of covergowns in the newborn nursery and masking in the labor room by staff or visitors have little justification as infection control measures (Larson, 1987).

Copp, Mailhot, Zalar, Slezak, and Copp (1986) studied the effectiveness of covergowns in protecting scrub suits worn by surgical personnel outside the operating room against bacterial contamination. Twenty subjects participated in four treatment regimens during their

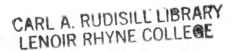

lunch breaks outside the operating room: (a) using covergowns over scrub suit; (b) wearing of the same scrub suit, unprotected by a covergown, throughout an entire working day; (c) changing into outdoor clothing for lunch and putting on a clean scrub suit after lunch; and (d) changing into outdoor clothing for lunch and donning the same scrub suit after lunch. The investigators found a protective effect of wearing covergowns for total bacterial colonization of the scrub suits as well as for counts of *Staphylococcus aureus* and concluded that the use of covergowns seemed to be protective. No attempt in this study was made to evaluate the effect of attire of surgical personnel on postoperative wound infection rates.

Two studies involving gloving practices have been reported recently. Roth and Whitbourne (1982) reported results of a small pilot study to assess the importance of closed versus open gloving technique. The gloving technique seemed to be of little importance bacteriologically. Larson, Wilder, and Laughon (1987) examined the effect of placing sterile petroleum jelly on hands prior to gloving, a practice sometimes followed by surgical nurses to reduce skin trauma. In 10 subjects who wore gloves for 15 minutes, 1 hour, and 4 hours, in successive tests, there were no significant differences in microbial growth on the hand randomly assigned to be covered with petroleum jelly compared to the other hand. The authors concluded that this seemed to be a safe practice, at least in the short term. However, long-term effects of this practice were not assessed.

Handwashing and Aseptic Technique.   Handwashing generally is accepted as the primary and most important strategy for reducing the risk of cross-infection (Centers for Disease Control, 1985; Semmelweis, 1861). Nursing research related to handwashing during the period reviewed was of two types: studies designed to describe the microorganisms present on hands and factors that affected the numbers and types of bacteria isolated from hands, and studies concerned with behavioral aspects of handwashing.

In a random sample of 103 hospital personnel and 50 members of the general population studied over a mean of 35 days (Larson, 1981), one or more of 22 species of gram-negative bacteria were carried persistently on the hands of 21% of nurses and physicians and 80% of controls. These same types of organisms were responsible for 21% of nosocomial infections in the study hospital (only correlation, not causation, was implied). The author concluded from this descriptive survey that such organisms are much more common on normal skin than generally thought. In a secondary analysis of these same data (Larson, 1984), it was determined that the type of soap, frequency of handwashing, and clinical unit were correlated significantly with numbers and types of organisms isolated. For example, nurses and physicians washing their hands more than eight times per day were less likely to be colonized with gram-negative bacteria and, if colonized, had significantly fewer organisms on their hands than those washing less than four times per day. A limitation of this finding was that handwashing frequency was determined by subject report and was not verified in observational studies. Additionally, it was reported that personnel working in obstetrics and nonpatient care areas had the greatest numbers of organisms on hands, and those working on neonatal and medical–surgical units had significantly lower numbers. It was not possible to determine whether such differences might have been explained by differences in handwashing practices.

Two investigators have examined the effect of ring wearing on hand flora. Jacobsen, Thiele, McCure, and Farrell (1985) used an experimental design with 10 student volunteers who conducted 256 sets of hand scrubs. For each subject, the first scrubs were conducted while wearing two to five rings and the rest of the scrubs, conducted at least 48 hours apart, were without rings. A standardized scrub protocol was used, and bacterial cultures were obtained before and after each scrub. Significantly higher counts were obtained in prescrub baseline counts on ringed hands, but no statistically significant differences between ringed and nonringed hands were noted after washing. The authors concluded that handwashing reduced the counts on ringed hands adequately. Two protocol concerns must be mentioned, however. First, the sequence of ringed and nonringed washes was not determined randomly, so that variables associated with sequence were uncontrolled (e.g., skill of the subject with the protocol). More importantly, nurses usually wash their hands for considerably shorter duration than 2 minutes. Would a shorter wash still have been effective in reducing the higher counts from the ringed hands? Thus, the fact that prescrub counts were significantly higher when rings were worn is still a concern.

Rozantals (1980) reported on the effect of wearing rings on hands that were gloved for 1 hour. The average bacterial count with rings was 647 colony-forming units, and without rings, 86. Unfortunately, there was no clear description of sampling methods, and no statistical analysis of results was reported. This sizable difference, nevertheless, is probably clinically important. Although these two studies together imply that ring wearing has an adverse effect on bacterial contamination of the hands, more definitive controlled and clinically applicable studies are indicated.

Behavioral aspects of handwashing and aseptic practices have been the focus of several other nursing studies. Recognizing that handwashing often is practiced suboptimally, Larson and Killien (1982) used a decision theory model in a survey of 193 nurses and physicians to identify factors influencing their handwashing behavior. Although frequent and infrequent washers did not differ significantly in their values regarding factors favoring handwashing, several deterrents to handwashing were identified. Individuals who washed infrequently, less than eight times per day, placed significantly more value on the detrimental effect of frequent washing on their own skin and were more concerned with the handwashing practices of their work colleagues than did individuals who washed frequently. A weakness of the study was that subject report of handwashing frequency was not verified by observation. The authors concluded that more emphasis should be placed on minimizing deterrents rather than on emphasizing the importance of handwashing.

Based on the results of this study, two subsequent studies were conducted to investigate further the influence of peer behavior on handwashing practices and to measure the detrimental effects of handwashing on the skin. In an experimental study in which an attending physician role model consistently washed his hands after patient examination, the handwashing behavior of other medical staff on his team was increased significantly when compared with a control team (Larson, 1985). It appeared that the handwashing behavior of a colleague could influence the practices of others. Unfortunately, however, the study was continued for only 2 months, so the long-term effect of this type of role model was not determined.

To address the problem of skin damage associated with frequent handwashing, a laboratory-based experiment using 52 female volunteers was conducted (Larson, Leyden, McGinley, Grove, & Talbot, 1986). Subjects washed their hands 24 times each day using a standardized protocol and one of five products: water alone, nonmedicated bar soap, or one of three antiseptic-containing products. Some damage to the stratum corneum occurred in all groups, but damage was not associated necessarily with those products used most frequently by health care personnel. Using objective physiologic measures of skin trauma with reported validity and reliability, it was possible to demonstrate that handwashing, with or without soap, did indeed cause skin trauma. The authors recommended that handwashing products be evaluated in terms of mildness and user comfort to minimize the importance of this deterrent to washing.

To determine the extent to which reported and observed handwashing behavior was correlated, an observational study on an oncology unit was conducted for two months (Larson, McGinley, Grove, Leyden, & Talbot, 1986). During 891 person-hours of observation, 986 handwashes by nursing and medical personnel were observed. Reported and observed practices were correlated only moderately. Physicians washed significantly less often but more thoroughly than nurses. The handwashing practices of individual nurses were found to vary significantly and were not associated necessarily with the extent of patient contact. Another investigator (Lawrence, 1983) administered a questionnaire regarding handwashing to hospitalized patients confined to bed. Eleven of 20 were not given opportunity for handwashing after toileting; 17 of the 20 never asked the nurse for assistance with handwashing, and they all reported handwashing after toileting at home.

Based on these studies of handwashing, it appears that nurses' hands are contaminated with microorganisms that are known to cause nosocomial infections and that their handwashing practices are influenced by a number of factors, including the harshness of soap and the behavior of their colleagues. There is urgent need, particularly in the wake of changes in practice such as increased gloving and the common practice of body substance isolation, for additional studies related to handwashing.

The most pressing research needed on this subject is for randomized clinical trials of antiseptic versus plain handwashing and the effects on rates of cross-infection. There are many difficulties associated with such clinical studies, including controlling potentially confounding variables, assuring compliance with study regimens over prolonged periods of time, obtaining adequate sample sizes, and obtaining sufficient funding for large, multicenter efforts. Because of these difficulties, such studies have not been done. The efficacy of handwashing in reducing risk of infection is, of course, the primary research question. Clearly, a second urgent research need is for behavioral studies that are addressed to issues of compliance of health care professionals with handwashing.

Compliance issues similar to those identified with handwashing have been noted also by investigators evaluating aseptic technique. Crow and Taylor (1983) observed 35 nurses in the surgical suite, noting infraction in surgical scrub procedures, room preparation, and handling of sterile equipment. Similarly, McLane, Chenelly, Sylwestrak, and Kirchhoff (1983) observed 34 nurses performing one of 22 clinical procedures such as bladder catheterization, oropharyngeal suctioning, or changing a dry sterile dressing. The majority of errors (89%) noted were failure to observe aseptic technique. Kasal (1985) surveyed 200 randomly selected members of The Association of Operating Room Nurses (AORN) in 119 hospitals. The 110 respondents were asked to identify and rank infractions in aseptic technique. For fewer than half of the infractions listed was there a consensus from respondents regarding whether the infractions were major or minor.

Patient Care Practices

Enteral/Parenteral Therapies.   In five recent nursing studies researchers have addressed infection issues related to breast milk, tube feeding, and intravascular therapy and monitoring. Crocker, Krey, Markovic, and Steffee (1986) prospectively compared bacterial contamination of refilled and prefilled enteral feeding systems when used according to standard protocols. A total of 57 days of feeding in 19 patients were studied; and formula was sampled at 0, 4, 8, 12, and 48 hours on 3 separate days for each patient. Approximately 60% of the 780 samples were contaminated. Microbial growth was greatest in reconstituted formulas, and there were no significant differences between canned formula and prefilled pouches. The greatest bacterial growth was present at the distal hub of the tubing. The authors concluded that prefilled bags delay bacterial contamination and that minimal manipulation of the enteral feeding system is desirable. Although the sample size was too small to correlate bacterial contamination with patient infections, enteral feedings do pose a risk of infection to patients, and this study provided data upon which to base guidelines for proper handling of enteral feeding systems.

Larson, Zuill, Zier, and Berg (1984) examined the bacteriologic content of breast milk expressed by 30 mothers for administration to their premature infants. These investigators were concerned about safe storage time for expressed milk as well as whether it was acceptable to allow mothers to express the milk at home and bring it to the clinical unit. A total of 120 breast milk samples were tested, 90 of which were obtained under nursing supervision in the hospital and 30 of which were expressed by the mothers at home. Milk samples were cultured at the time of expression and then after refrigeration for 24 and 48 hours.

There were no significant differences in colony counts between the three time intervals or between samples expressed at home and at the hospital. Based on these findings, the investigators concluded that it was safe to store refrigerated breast milk for up to 48 hours and to allow the mother to bring expressed milk from home. These findings served as the basis for development of the study unit's policy regarding storage of breast milk.

Josephson, Gombert, Sierra, Karanfil, and Tansino (1985) examined the relationship between contamination of intravenous (IV) fluid and the frequency of IV tubing replacement. In this well-controlled prospective clinical trial over an 11-month period, 219 3-day or longer courses of IV therapy were studied. Subjects receiving IV therapy were assigned randomly to 48-hour tubing changes or no tubing changes except when the entire IV system was changed. The average time that tubing was used was 1.8 days in the 48-hour group and 4.3 days in the no-change group. There were no significant differences in contamination of fluid (0.87% and 0.96% respectively) or in the cumulative probability of tubing surviving free of contamination (.988 and .087 respectively). The researchers concluded that it was safe to leave IV tubing in place for up to 4 days.

Addressing a different patient care practice related to hemodynamic monitoring, Yonkman and Hamory (1984) compared three methods of maintaining a sterile injectate system for cardiac output determination. A randomized crossover design was used to compare the closed loop injectate system, a capped syringe, and a double-bag system. Forty-five subjects were assigned randomly to one system, and then crossed over to an alternate. The investigators found a significant difference in bacterial colonization between the closed-loop method (0 out of 30) and each of the other two methods (6 out of 30, $p < .001$). The closed-loop method was also less costly and time consuming.

The final study dealing with parenteral therapy was a quasi-experimental inquiry designed to evaluate a program in which trained staff nurses in lieu of medical house staff or a centralized IV team maintained IV therapy on clinical units. Outcomes evaluated included phlebitis and infusion-related infections as well as costs and patient comfort. Among the 879 infusions in 707 patients studied, phlebitis rates decreased significantly on experimental units and increased slightly on control units when compared with baseline rates. On the other hand, bacterial colonization of IV devices occurred more often on experimental units, 19.4% versus 5.9%, $p < .01$, but there were no infections in either group. The authors concluded that such a decentralized program could be successful if it included a system of monitoring to assure compliance with written guidelines. A weakness of the study design was that although every effort was made to match experimental and control units, they might have varied on other factors that also could have influenced study results (Larson & Hargiss, 1984).

Respiratory Care. One controversy in nursing care of patients with tracheostomies has been whether sterile technique is necessary for tracheostomy care. Harris and Hyman (1984) examined this issue in a retrospective chart review of patients undergoing tracheostomy after head and neck surgery in 10 different hospitals. Using a rather sophisticated statistical procedure, charts of 209 patients who had received either sterile, clean, or "mixed" tracheostomy care were examined carefully for indications of pulmonary infection, using an investigator-developed rating tool. The authors found that use of the clean procedure was associated with the fewest postoperative infections. The several design problems in this study included the fact that, as in all retrospective studies, there was no control over group assignment of patients, it was not possible to determine whether the three treatment groups were comparable, it was difficult to differentiate between colonization of patients and true clinical infection, and the investigator-developed tool needed further reliability and validity testing. Nevertheless, the study provides at least enough preliminary data to justify an experimental design in which patients are assigned randomly to clean or sterile technique.

In another study, resuscitation bags were examined as a source of bacterial contamination (Thompson, Wilder, & Powner, 1985). In 12 bags in use for 24 hours, both the connection valve and the aerosol from the bags were sampled. Three-fourths of the valves and one-fourth of the aerosols were contaminated with organisms such as *Klebsiella, Pseudomonas,* and *Streptococcus pneumoniae.* The researchers made several recommendations that might reduce the risk of contamination. They suggested that the oxygen flow through the bag be discontinued when the bag is not in use, that the valves be cleaned frequently, and that the bags be enclosed in containers when not in use and be replaced every 24 hours. Further studies to assess the effectiveness of such measures in reducing levels of bacterial contamination seem warranted.

Nelsey (1986) reported a small study in which four mouth care procedures for the intubated patient were compared. Unfortunately, however, there was only one mouth care regimen, so the results of the study do not warrant further discussion here. An important finding was that the normal oral flora of all four patients had been replaced by coliforms within 48 hours of intubation. This emphasizes the urgent need for nursing research to assess various mouth care regimens to reduce the patient's risk of pulmonary infection.

Other Practices. Various innovations in patient beds have become available in recent years. These are designed to enhance skin integrity. Bolyard, Townsend, and Horan (1987) examined the potential for airborne contamination associated with one such bed, the air-fluidized bed. In 12 patients bedridden for at least 7 days, 2-minute air samples were taken at several specified sites with the patient first on a conventional bed and then on days 1, 5, 6, and 7 on an air-fluidized bed. Each patient's urine and skin lesions or groin were sampled also on days 5 and 7 to determine congruence between patient colonizing flora and organisms isolated from the air. There were no significant differences in any sampling results between conventional and air-fluidized beds. A strength of this study is that sampling conditions were controlled carefully to minimize effects of extraneous variables. The investigators wore gown, masks, and gloves during air sampling; a 30-minute settling period was required with the door closed before air samples in the room were taken, and talking and visitors within the room were minimized.

SUMMARY AND DIRECTIONS FOR FUTURE RESEARCH

The vast majority of the infection control nursing research conducted in the past decade has been concerned with nosocomial infections in hospitals and, hence, these investigators have addressed problems related to patient care practices, equipment, and procedures specific to that setting. In addition, a number of studies have been concerned with the behavioral aspects of infection control.

Future research in this field needs to be expanded in several ways. First, there is clear need for more research focused on the outcome of reduction in risk of infection. Risk of infection is the result of a number of interacting host, environmental, and microbial factors. Without carefully controlled prospective studies with large sample sizes, it is extremely difficult to infer a causal link between various nursing practices and risk of infection. The need for such clinical trials is particularly urgent to examine effectiveness of isolation precautions and the use of antimicrobial-containing versus plain soap for hand-washing and skin cleansing. Realistically, however, one cannot expect that many such studies will be attempted because of limitations of cost, time, and expertise, and because the study design problems are daunting. Nevertheless, it is essential that efficacious infection control practices be identified so that behavioral techniques can be applied to emphasize those practices shown to be most effective.

A second need for expansion of nursing research in infection control is in the area of study setting. While nosocomial infections occur in 5 to 10% of hospitalized patients, rates are even higher in extended care facilities, day care centers, and home care settings (Haley, Culver, White, Morgan, & Emori, 1985). Infection control research endeavors in these settings are just beginning and need expanding. For example, a postdoctoral nursing fellow currently is studying the effectiveness of an educational intervention related to handwashing and diapering in reducing the incidence of diarrhea in home day care centers, a setting that previously has received minimal attention. A major advantage in the field of infection control is that research endeavors have been traditionally undertaken by interdisciplinary teams. Nurses have an established and highly respected role in such team efforts; their clinical expertise and roles in effecting practice changes are an essential part of the practice of infection control.

REFERENCES

Albert, R. K., & Condie, F. (1981). Handwashing patterns in medical intensive care units. *New England Journal of Medicine, 304,* 1465–1466.
Bolyard, E. A., Townsend, R. R., & Horan, T. (1987). Airborne contamination associated with in-use air-fluidized beds: A descriptive study. *American Journal of Infection Control, 15,* 75–78.
Boxall, J., Orme, R. L. E., & Cruickshank, J. G. (1982). Shared care and infection in a special care baby unit. *Nursing Times, 78,* 1848–1850.
Campbell, V. G. (1987). Covergowns for newborn infection control? *MCN: American Journal of Maternal Child Nursing, 12* (1), 54.
Centers for Disease Control. (1985). *CDC guideline for handwashing and hospital environmental control.* Atlanta, GA: Author.
Cohen, I. B. (1984). Florence Nightingale. *Scientific American, 250,* 128–137.
Cooper, H. M. (1982). Scientific guidelines for conducting integrative research reviews. *Review of Educational Research, 52,* 291–302.

Copp, G., Mailhot, C. B., Zalar, M., Slezak, L., & Copp, A. J. (1986). Cover-gowns and the control of operating room contamination. *Nursing Research, 35,* 263–368.

Crocker, K. S., Krey, S. H., Markovic, M., & Steffee, W. P. (1986). Microbial growth in clinically used enteral delivery systems. *American Journal of Infection Control, 14,* 250–256.

Crow, S., & Taylor, E. (1983). Nurses compliance with aseptic technique. *Association of Operating Room Nurses Journal, 37,* 1066–1072.

Diers, D. (1979). *Research in nursing practice.* Philadelphia: Lippincott.

Donowitz, L. G. (1986). Failure of the overgown to prevent nosocomial infection in a pediatric intensive care unit. *Pediatrics, 77,* 35–38.

Duffy, M. E. (1985). A research appraisal checklist for evaluating nursing research reports. *Nursing & Health Care, 6,* 539–547.

Federal Register. (1987, October 30). Protection against occupational exposure to hepatitis B virus (HBV) and human immuno-deficiency virus. *52*(210), 41818–41823.

Forfar, J. O., & McCabe, A. F. (1958). Masking and gowning in nurseries for the newborn infant. *British Medical Journal, 1,* 76–79.

Gilmore, D. S., Montgomerie, J. Z., & Graham, I. E. (1986). Category 1, 2, 3, and 4: A procedure-oriented isolation system. *Infection Control, 7,* 263–267.

Haley, R. W. (1986). *Managing hospital infection control for cost-effectiveness.* Chicago: American Hospital Association.

Haley, R. W., Culver, D. H., White, J. W., Morgan, W. M., & Emori, T. G. (1985). The nationwide nosocomial infection rates. *American Journal of Epidemiology, 121,* 159–167.

Haley, R. W., Culver, D. H., White, J. W., Morgan, W. M., Emori, T. G., Munn, V. P., & Hooton, T. M. (1985). The efficacy of infection surveillance and control programs in preventing nosocomial infections in US hospitals. *American Journal of Epidemiology, 121,* 182–204.

Harris, R. B., & Hyman, R. B. (1984). Clean vs. sterile tracheotomy care and level of pulmonary infection. *Nursing Research, 33,* 80–91.

Hunter, M. A., & Williams, D. (1985). Mask wearing in the labor ward. *Midwives Chronicle and Nursing Notes, 98* (1164), 12–13.

Jackson, M. M., & Lynch, P. (1985). Isolation practices: A historical perspective. *American Journal of Infection Control, 13,* 21–31.

Jacobsen, G., Thiele, J. E., McCure, J. H., & Farrell, L. D. (1985). Handwashing, ring-wearing and number of microorganisms. *Nursing Research, 34,* 186–188.

Josephson, A., Gombert, M. E., Sierra, M. F., Karanfil, L. V., & Tansino, G. F. (1985). The relationships between intravenous fluid contamination and the frequency of tubing replacement. *Infection Control, 6,* 367–370.

Kasal, S. E. (1985). Infractions in aseptic technique. *Association of Operating Room Nurses Journal, 41,* 611–620.

Kowba, M. D., & Schwirian, P. M. (1985). Direct sibling contact and bacterial colonization in newborns. *Journal of Obstetric, Gynecologic, and Neonatal Nursing, 14,* 412–417.

Larson, E. (1981). Persistent carriage of gram-negative bacteria on hands. *American Journal of Infection Control, 9,* 112–119.

Larson, E. (1983). Compliance with isolation technique. *American Journal of Infection Control, 11,* 221–225.

Larson, E. (1984). Effects of handwashing agent, handwashing frequency, and clinical area on hand flora. *American Journal of Infection Control, 12,* 76–82.

Larson, E. (1985). One hand washes the other. *American Journal of Nursing, 85,* 1324.

Larson, E. L. (1987). Rituals and infection control: What works in the newborn nursery. *Journal of Obstetric, Gynecologic and Neonatal Nursing, 16,* 411–417.

Larson, E. L. (1988). Nursing research and AIDS. *Nursing Research, 31,* 60–62.

Larson, E., & Hargiss, C. (1984). A decentralized approach to maintenance of intravenous therapy. *American Journal of Infection Control, 12,* 177–186.

Larson, E., Hargiss, C. O., & Dyk, L. (1985). Effects of an expanded physical facility on nosocomial infections in a neonatal intensive care unit. *American Journal of Infection Control, 13,* 16–20.

Larson, E., & Killien, M. (1982). Factors influencing handwashing behavior of patient care personnel. *American Journal of Infection Control, 10,* 93–99.

Larson, E., Leyden, J. J., McGinley, K. J., Grove, G. L., & Talbot, G. H. (1986). Physiologic and microbiologic changes in skin related to frequent handwashing. *Infection Control, 7,* 59–63.

Larson, E., McGinley, K. J., Grove, G. L., Leyden, J. J., & Talbot, G. H. (1986). Physiologic, microbiologic, and seasonal effects of handwashing on the skin of health care personnel. *American Journal of Infection Control, 14,* 51–59.

Larson, E. L., Wilder, M. P., & Laughon, B. E. (1987). Microbiologic effects of emollient on gloved hands. *American Journal of Infection Control, 15,* 168–171.

Larson, E., Zuill, R., Zier, V., & Berg, B. (1984). Storage of human breast milk. *Infection Control, 5,* 127–130.

Lawrence, M. (1983). Patient hand hygiene—A clinical inquiry. *Nursing Times, 79*(22), 24–25.

Lynch, P., Jackson, M. M., Cummings, M. J., & Stamm, W. E. (1987). Rethinking the role of isolation practices of nosocomial infections. *Annals of Internal Medicine, 107,* 243–246.

McLane, C., Chenelly, S., Sylwestrak, M. L., & Kirchhoff, K. T. (1983). A nursing practice problem: Failure to observe aseptic technique. *American Journal of Infection Control, 11,* 178–182.

National Institutes of Health. (1987). Nursing research related to AIDS. *NIH Guide to grants and contracts, 16,* 1.

Nelsey, L. (1986). Mouthcare and the intubated patient—The aim of preventing infection. *Intensive Care Nursing, 1,* 187–193.

Nightingale, F. (1863). *Notes on hospitals* (3rd ed.). London: Longman, Green, Longman, Roberts, & Green.

Preston, G. A., Larson, E. L., & Stamm, W. E. (1981). The effect of private isolation rooms on patient care practices, colonization and infection in an intensive care unit. *American Journal of Medicine, 70,* 641–645.

Renaud, M. T. (1983). Effects of discontinuing cover gowns on a postpartal ward upon cord colonizations of the newborn. *Journal of Obstetric, Gynecologic and Neonatal Nursing, 12,* 399–401.

Roberts, J. E., Hammes, B., & Gundersen, J. (1986). Professional attire at delivery, effect on postpartum and neonatal infection. *Journal of Nurse-Midwifery, 31,* 16–19.

Rosenberg, C. E. (1979). Florence Nightingale on contagion: The hospital as moral universe. In C. E. Rosenberg (Ed.), *Healing and history* (pp. 116–136). New York: Science History Publications.

Roth, K. A., & Whitbourne, J. (1982). A pilot study of open and closed surgical gloving. *Association of Operating Room Nurses Journal, 36,* 571–576.

Rozantals, J. (1980). Keep it clean! *Nursing Mirror, 151* (Supplement, Oct. 9), x–xvi.

Semmelweis, I. F. (1861). *The etiology, the concept and the prophylaxis of childbed fever* (F. P. Murphy, trans.). Pest, Hungary: Hartleben's Verlag-Eppedition. (Republished by Classics of Medicine Library, Birmingham, England 1981).

Thompson, A. C., Wilder, B. J., & Powner, D. J. (1985). Bedside resuscitation bags: A source of bacterial contamination. *Infection Control, 6,* 231–232.

Wranesh, B. L. (1982). The effects of sibling visitation on bacterial colonization rate in neonates. *Journal of Obstetric, Gynecologic and Neonatal Nursing, 11,* 211–213.

Yonkman, C. A., & Hamory, B. H. (1984). Comparison of three methods of maintaining a sterile injectate system during cardiac output determinations. *American Journal of Infection Control, 12,* 276–281.

PART II

Research on Nursing Care Delivery

Chapter 6

Nursing Diagnosis

MI JA KIM
COLLEGE OF NURSING
UNIVERSITY OF ILLINOIS AT CHICAGO

CONTENTS

The progress of research on nursing diagnosis mirrors that of the acceptance of the concept and utility of nursing diagnosis by the profession. Inclusion of nursing diagnosis in the definition[1] of nursing in the American Nurses' Association Social Policy Statement (1980, p. 9) and increasing use of nursing diagnosis by practicing nurses have propelled the acceptance of the concept by the profession in general. As in an earlier *Annual Review of Nursing Research* chapter on nursing diagnosis

[1] Nursing is the diagnosis and treatment of human responses to actual or potential health problems.

(Gordon, 1985), there continues to be a limited number of studies in this area, particularly when only publications in refereed research journals are considered. Because of its content or specific nature, most of the research on nursing diagnosis has been presented at the biennial National Conferences on Classification of Nursing Diagnoses and, subsequently, published in the *Proceedings* (Gebbie, 1976; Gebbie & Lavin, 1975; Hurley, 1986; Kim, McFarland, & McLane, 1984; Kim & Moritz, 1982; McLane, 1987). This trend continued until the mid-1980s, when an increasing number of articles began to appear in nursing journals and books.

Research articles published in the *Proceedings* of seven National Conferences on Classification of Nursing Diagnoses were reviewed by a panel of researchers using a process similar to that in refereed research journals. The major difference was that only abstracts, not full-length manuscripts, were reviewed for acceptance. Because articles published in the *North American Nursing Diagnosis Association* (NANDA)[2] *Proceedings* are generally unknown to nurses at large and are not retrievable readily by a conventional library citation system, research articles on nursing diagnoses are one of the best-kept secrets in nursing research. The purpose of this chapter is to present a critical review of research articles published on nursing diagnoses. Research articles published during the period of January 1973 to April 1987 were retrieved by MEDLINE search; a manual search was conducted on all volumes of NANDA *Proceedings* published during this period. Only those papers that dealt with general research methodologies for nursing diagnosis research and research articles that focused on identification and validation of nursing diagnoses are included in this review. Articles from the NANDA *Proceedings* were limited to those that were presented in the formal paper presentation sessions of the conferences.

Three reasons compelled the choice of these three types of articles for this chapter. First, introduction of major research methodologies for validation of nursing diagnoses would facilitate the conduct of nursing diagnosis research. Second, these articles constitute the bulk of research articles in the field. Third, these articles provide perhaps the most needed information for research and the development of nursing diagnoses. Hence, much attention is given to the methods and the substance of the study so as to benefit both researchers and clinicians. Because of multiple articles and limited space, the discussion is

[2] Previously called National Conference Group on Classification of Nursing Diagnosis.

limited to critical points only, and general remarks are made to reflect groups of articles.

The first section of this chapter is devoted to research methodologies for the validation of nursing diagnoses. This is followed by discussion of research for identification of nursing diagnoses and clinical validation studies of nursing diagnoses.

RESEARCH METHODOLOGIES FOR VALIDATION OF NURSING DIAGNOSES

The three models proposed by Gordon and Sweeney (1979) for identification and validation of nursing diagnoses were the most frequently cited and used research methods. The models are the Retrospective Identification Model, the Clinical Model, and the Nurse Validation Model.

In the Retrospective Identification Model, the accumulated clinical experience and knowledge of nurses are utilized for identification and validation of nursing diagnoses. In the Clinical Model, diagnoses are identified and validated by nurses' direct observation of patient behaviors. The Nurse Validation Model can be applied to clinically tested or identified diagnoses. In this model, nurse subjects observe patients to determine if the preidentified defining characteristics (DCs) occur as a cluster in a sufficient number of cases. Given the broad scope of these methodologies and the early stage of research on nursing diagnosis in the late 1970s and early 1980s, the use of these models by numerous investigators is understandable.

Fehring (1986) modified the Gordon and Sweeney (1979) models and proposed two practical models: Diagnostic Content Validity (DCV) Model and Clinical Diagnostic Validity (CDV) Model, both of which provide quantifiable evidence for validity. Users of a DCV Model employ retrospective evidence from the perspective of experts on the characteristics of a given diagnostic label, whereas users of the CDV Model utilize prospective evidence on the characteristics from a clinical perspective. Explicit steps and the equation for CDV scoring (Fehring, 1986) have been used by several researchers for validation studies, as is presented later in this chapter.

Other research methods to identify and validate DCs of nursing diagnoses are Q methodology (Kerlinger, 1973), used by Lackey (1986) and Lawson and Lackey (1986); and the Delphi technique, used by Shoemaker (1984) and Frenn, Jacobs, Lee, Sanger, and Strong (1987). Also, Lo and Kim (1986) described a method to test construct validity of Sleep Pattern Disturbance. Three phases were involved: (a) generation of common DCs of Sleep Pattern Disturbance by a comprehensive literature review; (b) rating of DCs by master's- and doctorally-prepared nurse experts; and (c) direct clinical assessment of patients with medical–surgical problems for validation of DCs of Sleep Pattern Disturbance. These approaches may serve as guides for other research with a similar purpose.

IDENTIFICATION OF NURSING DIAGNOSES

Studies to identify nursing diagnoses in diverse groups of patients have varied in sophistication of design and presentation of findings. Many investigators aimed to identify both DCs and etiologies of nursing diagnoses. Two overall observations can be made of these articles. First was the range and average number of nursing diagnoses per patient found by investigators. Gebbie (1976) reported 3.97 diagnoses per patient, whereas 6.6 and 6.4 were reported by Jones (1982a, 1982b) respectively, and 5.0 by Gould (1983). The widest range of diagnoses was 1 to 16 per patient (Jones, 1982b). Second was the question raised by investigators as to whether or not the patient problem terminologies used by practicing nurses were similar to those of NANDA. Such questions can be noted particularly in the early years of NANDA, when affirmation or identification of different terminologies received more attention.

Two major methods were utilized in the identification of nursing diagnosis research: (a) questionnaire survey and (b) chart/care plan review. Research reports utilizing each of these methods are reviewed below.

Questionnaire Survey

Gebbie (1976) presented results of a survey of 28 agencies to identify nursing diagnoses that were used in assessing patient behaviors. She reported 2,338 nursing diagnoses from 588 patients and found that

81% of the nursing diagnoses were related directly to those identified at the First National Conference on Classification of Nursing Diagnoses. The average number of nursing diagnoses was 3.97 per patient. Castle (1982) found 650 nursing diagnoses with 1,442 DCs from 1 month of clinical study on 33 patients who were in an intensive care unit. The range of nursing diagnoses per patient was 1 to 9. Jones (1982a) found 613 nursing diagnoses during 93 nurse–client encounters with a mean of 6.6 nursing diagnoses per client. In another study, Jones (1982b) reported 2,517 nursing diagnoses from 393 nurse–client encounters; the average number of nursing diagnoses was 6.4 per client, with a range of 1 to 16. Fifty-seven master's- or baccalaureate-prepared nurses generated these nursing diagnoses.

Vincent (1985a, 1985b) used a diagnostic criteria questionnaire survey method to describe the frequency of DCs for the nursing diagnosis Ineffective Coping, Individual. One thousand clinical nurse specialists were selected randomly from a pool of 1,183; each specialist received a 5-point graphic rating scale in which each DC of the diagnosis was listed. Anxiety and Reported Life Stress were new DCs added to the 11 DCs generated by NANDA (Kim & Moritz, 1982). An open-ended question was added for participants to write in other characteristics as necessary. They were instructed to consider a hypothetical sample of 100 clients with Ineffective Coping and indicate how frequently this population exhibited the specific signs and symptoms of the diagnosis. The Cronbach's alpha was 0.740 for the instrument with the final study sample ($N = 513$). Anxiety and Reported Life Stress had the highest median score of 5. Inability to Problem Solve was reported as "nearly always to frequently" present by 82% of the clinical nurse specialists. However, one might question whether Anxiety and Reported Life Stress are DCs or etiologies of Ineffective Coping.

Baas and Allen (1985) proposed a new nursing diagnosis, Memory Error. Two hundred and twenty-four men and women taking daily, long-term medication responded to a questionnaire that included two scenarios of Memory Error (one depicting a schedule error, the other an episodic error). Scenarios were used to decrease potential defensive behavior from subjects. Subjects were asked if they experienced the same problem as the person in the story. Three types of subjects participated in the study: patients from an outpatient cardiac rehabilitation phase II program ($n = 27$); members of support groups for epilepsy, diabetes, and Parkinsonism ($n = 45$); and college students enrolled in an introductory psychology course ($n = 152$). Most respondents reported making both types of Memory Error. Ninety-four percent reported that they had experienced schedule errors, and 83% reported making episodic errors. Even though currently four other nursing diagnoses describe a condition of a patient who is noncompliant with a prescribed regimen, Baas and Allen presented an argument for inclusion of Memory Error as a nursing diagnosis. The other nursing diagnoses are: Noncompliance, Knowledge Deficit, Health Maintenance Impairment, and Altered Thought Process. The authors argued that none of these diagnoses adequately incorporate the problem of memory and having this as a separate diagnosis would yield different intervention and evaluation methods. However, it is conceivable that Memory Error could serve as an etiology for those four nursing diagnoses. Reliance on self-report, the global nature of assessment, and lack of cluster of signs and symptoms for this nursing diagnosis are other aspects of the study that require further examination.

Chart/Care Plan Review

In nine studies, chart ($n = 8$) and care plan ($n = 1$) review were used as methods to identify nursing diagnoses and DCs. Seven studies dealt with nursing diagnoses of patients in the hospital setting, and two addressed nursing diagnoses in community nursing practice.

In a study of patients with obstetric and gynecological problems ($N = 104$) who were referred to the Visiting Nurses Association (VNA) by a hospital, McKeehan and Gordon (1982) found 567 nursing diagnoses recorded, 43% of which were NANDA-approved nursing diagnoses. Alteration in Parenting was the most frequently identified nursing diagnosis.

Retrospective chart review was done by Silver, Halfmann, McShane, Hunt, and Nowak (1984) to identify nursing diagnoses and substantiating indicators in 377 adult medical–surgical patients. A total of 1,344 diagnostic labels with multiple indicators were found. These labels were classified into 16 major categories by five national experts in nursing diagnosis. Alteration in Comfort: Pain was the most frequent nursing diagnosis: 33% of its indicators were subjective data.

Suhayda and Kim (1984) conducted a retrospective chart audit on 25 medical and 25 surgical intensive care charts to evaluate the documentation of the nursing process in critical care and to identify the most commonly documented patient problems, actions, and patient outcomes. Twenty percent of the charts were selected randomly and reexamined independently by a medical–surgical clinical nurse specialist using the same tool. Interrater agreement was 93%. There was no documented evidence that problem identification was linked to nursing action or patient outcome. Furthermore, patient problems were described in unclustered and unrelated pieces of assessment data. Hence, patient problems identified in this paper were based on the investigators' inferences of the nurses' descriptions. The two most frequently identified patient problems were Impaired Ventilatory/Circulatory Function and Pain/Discomfort. Documented interventions followed problem categories, although their relationships were not always clear. Nursing interventions were documented in only 81% of the cases describing patient problems.

One overall concern with chart review studies is that the data generated from this method are not valid and reliable unless nurses recorded their professional practice with the understanding and implementation of the concept of nursing diagnosis. Some investigators failed to mention this aspect, leaving readers to question the outcomes of the studies.

Recognizing the weakness of a one-group design, Janken and Reynolds (1987) conducted a retrospective comparative chart audit on 631 patients aged 60 and older to identify DCs of Falls. Incident reports and charts of 331 patients who fell between July 1, 1982 and March 31, 1984 provided data for the Fall category. The 24-hour period preceding the fall as recorded in these documents was audited. The No-Fall category data were obtained by means of a simple random sample drawn from charts of patients who did not fall and who met the age and hospital-stay criteria stated above. The charts of the No-Fall group were audited once on a randomly selected day of hospital stay. Charts of both categories were audited for the period of the first 24 hours of hospitalization. Results of a stepwise regression analysis revealed seven variables that significantly added to the total variance in both the admission day and fall/random day equations: confusion, building structure, sleeplessness, decreased mobility of the lower extremities, incontinence, general weakness, and employment status. The authors suggested that confusion, impaired mobility of the lower extremities, alcohol abuse, incontinence, and being elderly were appropriate DCs for the diagnosis Potential for Fall.

Munns (1985) conducted a retrospective chart audit to identify and validate DCs and critical indicators for the nursing diagnosis Potential for Violence. The sample consisted of two groups of patients identified as violent or potentially violent in a neuropsychiatric unit ($n = 20$) and long-term care ($n = 10$) Veteran's Administration hospital.

The most frequent primary psychiatric diagnosis for all subjects was schizophrenia (66%). Charts were reviewed for a 5-day period prior to the incident of violence; DCs for Potential for Violence were compared to those 5 days of notes to see if nurses and other health professionals recorded any cues before the incident occurred. Content validity of the tool was established by literature review and input from expert practitioners.

The DCs that occurred in 33% of the cases were defined as valid; those occurring in 50% or more of the cases were defined as critical. Based on these criteria, seven of the DCs were considered valid and five critical. Two areas of concern are raised in this study. The first is the question of the validity and reliability of the data because the concept of nursing diagnosis was not integrated sufficiently into nursing practice, and the data were also from other health professionals' records. The second concern is the use of 33% and 50% of the cases; these percentages are too low for the determination of valid and critical DCs.

Creason, Pogue, Nelson, and Hoyt (1985) used 84 nursing care plans developed by registered nurse (RN) students who were enrolled in a rehabilitation nursing practicum. They asked two questions: (a) what is the frequency of the nursing diagnosis Impaired Physical Mobility; and (b) what are the patterns of the etiologies and DCs in this diagnosis? An excellent feature of this study was that each etiology and DC was defined operationally by the investigators. Thirty-four (40.5%) nursing care plans that used the diagnosis of Impaired Physical Mobility in the accepted format of Problem–Etiology–Signs and Symptoms were reviewed. The cumulative interrater reliability was 0.97. Interrater reliability for etiology was 0.98 and 0.96 for DCs when researchers evaluated 10 randomly chosen nursing care plans. A total of 94 DCs were identified, and 75% of these were classified into four broad categories in descending order: inability to perform self-care; decreased muscle strength, control, or mass; other functional alterations; and limited range of motion. An average of two etiologic statements per diagnosis was found. Medical diagnoses were used frequently as etiologies, as was the case in previous studies (Dougherty, 1985; Kim et al., 1982). The question they raised about Self-Care Deficit as a more appropriate diagnosis than Impaired Physical Mobility was an interesting point that deserves further consideration in delineating nursing diagnosis from etiology.

Martin (1982) reported a classification of client problems developed by the VNA of Omaha. Community nurses made two to three home visits to 338 families newly admitted to VNA care. Client problems were categorized into individual or family health problems, with further delineations as actual or potential. Each client problem had descriptions including signs and symptoms, risk factors, etiology, and laboratory tests. Four domains with 49 problem names and corresponding descriptions were reported: environmental, psychosocial, physiological, and health behaviors. This classification system frequently is used by community nurses, but it does not contain the term nursing diagnosis.

To identify the problem statements used by community health nurses and to compare them with the classification system of NANDA, Baldwin and Lueckenotte (1986) reviewed 150 records from three health departments. Of the 472 problem statements identified, only 9 (2%) were judged nursing diagnoses as defined by NANDA. This study demonstrated the need for a standardized diagnostic system in community health nursing.

CLINICAL VALIDATION OF NURSING DIAGNOSES

There were basically two types of studies with a focus on the clinical validation of nursing diagnoses. The first deals with identification/validation of nursing diagnoses in a group of patients with a common health problem; the second type was the validation of one or more individual nursing diagnoses with DCs, etiologies, and interventions. Studies that were aimed at identifying critical indicators generally had two major approaches. The first was the use of a Clinical Diagnostic Validity (CDV) score (Fehring, 1986) of 0.5 or greater, and the other was the use of the mean or median score (Lo & Kim, 1986: McFarland & Naschinski, 1985; Nicoletti, Reitz, & Gordon, 1982; Voith & Smith, 1985; York, 1985) as the cutoff point.

Research on individual diagnoses was categorized according to physiological, psychophysiological, and cognitive–perceptual domains. Whereas this classification schema was neither comprehensive nor mutually exclusive, these groupings were chosen for convenience of presentation and were developed on the basis of the articles reviewed in this section only. Studies that dealt with groups of diagnoses are presented first, followed by individual diagnoses according to aforementioned categories.

Validation Studies with Groups of Nursing Diagnoses

Nursing diagnoses in patients with chronic illness, multiple sclerosis, and cardiovascular disorders were studied by several investigators. Utilizing human need and motivation theories as the framework for health assessment and formation of nursing diagnoses, Hoskins, McFarlane, Rubenfeld, Walsh, and Schreier (1986) examined 169 adults with a medical diagnosis of chronic illness in order to determine nursing diagnoses. Five master's-prepared nurses interviewed 11 subjects over a period of 4 months. Interrater reliability of the interviews was 91%. This was followed by a clinical phase and a validation phase. Fifty-one diagnoses were identified. Six diagnoses were identified in more than 50% of the sample. In descending order, these were: Potential for Nutritional Deficiency (79%); Interference with Activity/Mobility: Pain (64%); Obesity (58%); Threatened Safety: Rats, Roaches, Pests (55%); Impaired Sleep Pattern (54%); and Potential for Eye/Vision Alterations (54%).

Gould (1983) examined 15 adult subjects with multiple sclerosis using Gordon's functional assessment tool, the diagnostic categories by the National Conference Group (Kim & Moritz, 1982), and other nursing diagnoses. Twenty-five nursing diagnoses were found in these subjects, with a range of 3 to 7, and an average of 5 nursing diagnoses per patient. Self-Care Deficit was found in 11 of 15 subjects (73%) and Self-Esteem Disturbance in 10 subjects (67%). Others were Potential Ineffective Family Coping: Compromised (47%), Sleep Disturbance (33%), and Social Isolation (33%). The major etiology for Self-Esteem Disturbance was altered body image; for Self-Care Deficit it was generalized weakness; for Social Isolation it was impaired mobility; and for Potential Ineffective Family Coping it was physical exhaustion of significant other.

In a structured survey of 76 RNs, Metzger and Hiltunen (1987) provided a list of ten NANDA-approved nursing diagnoses and asked these nurses to recall, from their most recent clinical experience, a representative sample of clients who had these diagnoses. Subjects were asked to rate the DCs of these diagnoses on a 5-point scale (5 = very characteristic to 1 = not characteristic). A weighted ratio was calculated for each DC using the DCV method (Fehring, 1986). Those cues with ratios greater than or equal to 0.75 were considered critical; those with a ratio less than 0.75 but greater than 0.50 were considered supporting characteristics. Limited space does not permit presentation of all defining characteristics of these ten nursing diagnoses. Readers are encouraged to review Tables 1 and 2 (pp. 148 to 150) in the Metzger and Hiltunen (1987) article.

Major strengths of the above studies were the use of a theoretical framework and master's-prepared clinical nurse experts. Using computers for validation of nursing diagnoses (Hoskins et al., 1986); and a weighted ratio of 0.75 as a cutoff point for determining critical defining characteristics (Metzger & Hiltunen, 1987) are other positive aspects of the studies.

Several studies were done to examine nursing diagnoses in cardiovascular patients. Kim and colleagues (1982, 1984) studied 158 adults with cardiovascular disorders to identify and validate nursing diagnoses in cardiovascular patients. Four cardiovascular clinical nurse specialists and 18 professional staff nurses from two hospitals participated in the study. All patients were assessed directly by staff nurses using a structured assessment guide. Thirty-eight of these patients were selected randomly and reassessed independently by clinical nurse specialists within 6 hours following the initial assessment by the staff nurse in order to validate the content of nursing diagnoses identified by the staff nurse and to establish reliability of the nursing diagnoses. From these 38 paired patient assessments, 36 different nursing diagnoses were identified and validated by both staff nurses and clinical nurse specialists. It is regrettable, however, that the authors were not able to establish validity and reliability of the DCs of each nursing diagnosis because of small sample size ($N = 158$).

Validation Studies with Individual Nursing Diagnoses

Physiological. Four major physiological nursing diagnoses that were studied by several investigators are Decreased Cardiac Output, Inadequate Coronary Artery Disease Risk Factor Modification, Ineffective Airway Clearance, and Ineffective Breathing Pattern. It is interesting to note that in all studies researchers addressed the issue of domain of nursing practice as it relates to these physiological nursing diagnoses. Most investigators reported that these diagnoses are within the scope of nursing practice because the majority of nursing interventions for these diagnoses were found to be independent. Dougherty (1985) and Dalton (1985) conducted clinical studies to validate the etiology and/or DCs of Decreased Cardiac Output. Dougherty used medical records of 20 patients with congestive heart failure and 13 patients with cardiogenic shock along with patient assessments and interviews with the medical and nursing staff. Most data were directly from nurses' notes written in narrative form.

Dougherty (1985) found the majority of etiologies to be medical diagnoses. Comparison made between NANDA categories and Dougherty's study in terms of DCs is instructive and useful. However, it is interesting to note that she listed DCs according to disease groups rather than the nursing diagnosis Decreased Cardiac Output. Furthermore, chest pain, which is suggested as a new DC for Decreased Cardiac Output, may be an etiology associated with myocardial infarction and coronary artery disease.

Because nurses were not using nursing diagnoses in Dougherty's (1985) study, a question can be raised about the validity of the inference statement, Decreased Cardiac Output. If nurses did not specify the nursing diagnosis, isolated signs and symptoms dispersed in the narrative (form) charting do not by themselves lead to the nursing diagnosis Decreased Cardiac Output. Additional confirmation by nurses' own documentation of nursing diagnosis would have strengthened the study. However, one should note that Dougherty's (1985) attempt was to validate DCs identified by NANDA.

Dalton (1985) used VNA discharge records to identify DCs of Decreased Cardiac Output. A strength of the study was that nurses in the VNA unit had been using nursing diagnosis for 5 years before the study was conducted. However, lack of actual patient validation was a weakness of the study. Conclusions drawn by Dalton (1985) and Dougherty (1985) about the use of Decreased Cardiac Output as a nursing diagnosis were quite interesting. Based on negative comments made by three clinical nurse specialists, Dalton (1985) raised questions regarding the usefulness of this diagnosis. Dougherty (1985), however, asserted that this diagnosis is within the realm of nursing practice by reporting that 77% of nursing interventions were considered to be independent by both nurses and physicians. This finding also was supported by the studies of Wessel and Kim (1984), who reported that 65% of nursing interventions for Decreased Cardiac Output were classified as independent nursing interventions. In addition, Hubalik and Kim (1984) showed that most of the NANDA diagnostic labels, including Decreased Cardiac Output, were within the scope of nursing practice and all were relevant to nursing interventions.

Burke, Gabriel, Fischer, and Zemke (1986) studied types and frequency of nursing diagnoses, DCs, and common nursing interventions for subjects admitted to a phase II cardiac rehabilitation program. Three cardiac rehabilitation nurse clinicians assessed 29 subjects during 6 to 12 weeks of the rehabilitation program. Careful attention was given to definitions, description of the program, and validity and reliability of the data collection instrument. Two nursing diagnoses were found: Inadequate Coronary Artery Disease Risk Factor Modification (100%) and Decreased Cardiac Output (14%). The investigators noted that 73% of the outcome criteria for these nursing diagnoses were achieved by the participants. Nursing interventions for both nursing diagnoses had many independent activities, which investigators noted as an indication that these diagnoses are within the realm of nursing practice.

Kim and colleagues (1982, 1984), Wessel and Kim (1984), Hubalik and Kim (1984), Dougherty (1985), and Dalton (1985) addressed a common question: Are physiological diagnoses truly nursing diagnoses? As reported earlier, these researchers demonstrated that physiological nursing diagnoses, including Decreased Cardiac Output, are within the scope of nursing practice, since the majority of nursing interventions were found to be independent. As Dalton reported, there are nurses who disagree with such findings, but such disagreements are bound to exist for any diagnosis.

York (1985) conducted a two-phase study to identify critical DCs of Ineffective Airway Clearance and Ineffective Breathing Pattern. In phase I, 10 nurses who worked in an acute-care respiratory unit rated the appropriateness of DCs for these two nursing diagnoses. Test–retest (interval not specified) results indicated that the tool was reliable. In phase II, the investigator reviewed 11 nursing care plans, which included respiratory nursing diagnoses made by a nurse regularly assigned to the respiratory unit. In the care plans, nurses noted presence or absence of DCs as well as etiologies for these diagnoses. Cough and sputum appeared as DCs for Ineffective Airway Clearance in 100% of the sample. Four additional DCs that were present in 91% of the sample were: dyspnea/shortness of breath (SOB), tachypnea, abnormal or decreased breath sounds, and ronchi/wheezes. Dyspnea/SOB was present in 100% of the sample for Ineffective Breathing Pattern, and abnormal blood gases in 91% of the sample, followed by accessory muscle use. Defining characteristics with such high incidence (91 to 100%) deserve to be considered critical ones for respective diagnoses.

Other physiological nursing diagnoses investigated were Constipation, Impaired Skin Integrity, and Urinary Retention. McShane and McLane (1985) validated the diagnosis of Constipation using the Gordon and Sweeney (1979) nurse-validation model. Following an in-depth literature review, the authors developed a checklist-type instrument that was used by 35 nurses in 10 agencies. One hundred and thirty instances of Constipation were recorded, and the data were used for further revision of the items. The authors reported, however, that they abandoned the nurse-validation model because of staff nurse resistance in completing the instrument and the limited amount of data used by them to make a diagnosis.

McShane and McLane (1985) also developed a parallel instrument to gather data from the clients' perspective. This tool was pilot-tested by 14 persons who lived in a long-term care facility. This was followed by a descriptive study in which 20 subjects living in a senior citizen's building were interviewed regarding bowel elimination practices. Data from this step were used for item revision and to derive a conceptual scheme for the variables of interest.

For empirical validation of diagnostic indicators, the investigators (McShane & McLane, 1985) collected data from 300 adult clients. It is not clear whether a questionnaire or interview was used for this step. Twenty-two DCs were identified by the respondents, but the authors reported that additional clinical studies were needed to identify critical DCs. It is regrettable that they could not identify critical DCs even after these multistep procedures.

Cattaneo and Lackey (1987) conducted a study to identify and validate DCs of Impaired Skin Integrity. Forty-two randomly selected enterostomal therapists from 11 regions of the United States responded to the Objects Content Test questionnaire (Hartley, 1970). A panel of five nurse experts validated the presence or absence of DCs. The 31 items that were identified from this step were subjected to a second questionnaire, which was completed by the same nurses who participated in the earlier step. Twenty-five of the 42 nurses returned the questionnaire. There was 90% agreement between the nurse experts and the enterostomal therapist respondents on the terms and phrases defining Impaired Skin Integrity.

To establish content validity of the nursing diagnosis Urinary Retention, Voith and Smith (1985) sent a questionnaire to nurses who worked in units where these diagnoses were prevalent. Nurses were asked to recall those patients who had this diagnosis, to confirm or reject signs and symptoms of Urinary Retention, and to rank from 1 (little relationship) to 5 (strong relationship) the degree of association of signs and symptoms and etiologic factors for the diagnosis of Urinary Retention. Items with values greater than 4.0 were termed critical. Fifty-three nurses responded to the questionnaire. Forty-eight percent perceived themselves as knowledgeable in the area of nursing diagnosis.

Distention, small frequent voidings, no urine output, sensation of bladder fullness, and dribbling were found to be critical indicators.

Some of the major etiological factors were weak sensory or motor impulses and strictures and flaccid bladder. Even though the authors presented critical indicators with a convincing criterion score of 4 or greater, the validity of the results can be questioned when one considers that only 48% of the nurse respondents felt they were knowledgeable about the topic of nursing diagnosis. However, it is possible that these nurses knew about urinary retention problems per se but not the concept of nursing diagnosis.

Psychophysiological. Although other diagnoses may fit very well into this category, only one study is presented under this heading. Guzzetta and Forsyth (1979) carried out a study in which five patients in a critical care unit were assessed in order to develop nursing diagnoses and etiologies for the Psychophysiologic Stress response. They used a biopsychosocial history and physical assessment. The anxiety part of the Sgroi, Holland, and Solkoff (1970) Anxiety-Depression Scale (A-D Scale) was used to assess anxiety. Data were collected from the patient, family, patient's history, physical examination, chart, care plan, and health team members to determine specific physiological, psychological, environmental, or sociocultural stressors, as well as psychophysiologic parameters and characteristics of stress. Observations were made of each patient in the critical care unit shortly after transfer to another unit, and again shortly before hospital discharge. Data were classified into four levels of stress according to a total psychophysiologic stress score (PPSS): low, moderate, high, and extreme. Physiologic and environmental factors were primary stressors during the critical care unit stay; psychologic and sociocultural factors were primary stressors shortly after transfer from the critical care unit and before discharge to home. The PPSS scores were highest during the critical care unit stay. Some physiologic parameters were found to be more substantive and sensitive than others: heart rate, dysrhythmias, blood pressure, respiratory rate, nausea/vomiting, and pupil size. There were no observable clusters of signs and symptoms when subjects were compared. This finding raises a question as to whether the term *psychophysiologic stress* satisfies the definition of nursing diagnosis, because it does not have a cluster of signs and symptoms as a nursing diagnosis usually would have (Gordon, 1982).

Cognitive-Perceptual. Twelve nursing diagnoses that belong to the cognitive perceptual category were studied. These diagnoses are: (a) Anxiety; (b) Altered Levels of Awareness in Significant Others; (c) Impaired Communication; (d) Non-compliance; (e) Knowledge Deficit; (f) Maternal Attachment; (g) Parenting Alteration; (h) Powerlessness;

(i) Self-Concept Alteration; (j) Disturbance in Self-Esteem; (k) Altered Body Image; and (l) Adolescent Identity Confusion. Note that the diagnoses Altered Levels of Awareness in Significant Others, Maternal Attachment, and Adolescent Identity Confusion have not been approved by NANDA. These diagnoses were included because each one was stated explicitly as a nursing diagnosis in these papers, and research on these nursing diagnoses meets the criteria specified for this chapter.

Fadden, Fehring, and Kenkel-Rossi (1987) conducted a study to validate the nursing diagnosis Anxiety using the clinical validation model of Gordon and Sweeney (1979). Ninety-one adult medical–surgical patients who were diagnosed as anxious by staff nurses received the state-anxiety component of Spielberger's State/Trait-Anxiety Inventory (Spielberger, Gorsuch, & Lushene, 1970). Forty-nine patients who had state-anxiety scores above 45 were assessed by two clinical specialists who examined the patients independently for each DC of anxiety. Data were analyzed by quantifying and ranking the frequency of observed characteristics from each specialist and by calculating the weighted interrater reliability ratio for each DC using Fehring's formula for CDV model (1986). None of the DCs reached a CDV score of 0.50 or greater, which indicates that no DC emerged as the critical indicator.

In both studies (Fadden et al., 1987; Guzzetta & Forsyth, 1979) researchers addressed the same diagnosis, Anxiety, using different tools. Neither presented a cluster of indicators for the diagnosis. Although Guzzetta and Forsyth emphasized that the A-D scale was clinically useful, it appeared that Anxiety was subsumed in the concept of Psychophysiologic Stress. However, the investigators' attempt to quantify different levels of stress is laudable and could be refined further to increase clinical sensitivity. The result of Fadden et al.'s (1987) study raised questions about the use of the criterion of a CDV score of 0.5 (Fehring, 1986) as a demarcation for critical indicators. One wonders if 0.5 might be too high, although other studies (Norris & Kunes-Connell, 1987) have used a higher score for a similar purpose.

To identify DCs for the nursing diagnosis of Altered Levels of Awareness in significant others, a panel of five experts (Group A) were mailed 102 cards that contained a list of 102 behaviors and feelings to Q-sort (Lawson & Lackey, 1986). Panelists were asked to rank the behaviors and feelings that were important in determining the diagnosis, Altered Levels of Awareness related to psychological impact. They were instructed to recall an emergency situation with a loved one and to complete the instrument regarding their feelings at the time of the incident. This activity was repeated in 1 week. The correlation coefficient for the total scores for the first and second administration of the instrument for each subject was 0.77. Cronbach's alpha was 0.85, but it was not clear whether this was for the second time only or both. The majority of the DCs were concerned with alteration in thinking, disturbed time sense, changes in emotional expressions, perceptual distortions, and body image changes.

McFarland and Naschinski (1985) conducted a study to identify and validate etiologic factors and DCs for Impaired Communication in adult psychiatric clients. Twenty-five nurses with master's or doctoral degrees in nursing and with a minimum of 2 years experience in psychiatric nursing responded to a survey tool and indicated their opinion as to whether each etiology and DC was relevant for the diagnosis. In addition, five nurses observed one client experiencing Impaired Communication for a total of 5 hours using a client observation tool developed for the diagnosis of impaired communication. Eleven etiologies received greater than 80% support by the respondents, and 25 DCs received greater than 68% support. It was not clear why the authors used different levels of support for etiologies and DCs.

To identify etiologies and DCs of Noncompliance and to describe nurses' perceptions of the importance of these etiologies and DCs in making the diagnosis of Noncompliance, 22 registered nurses who actively worked with patients whom they identified as noncompliant participated in a study by Ryan and Falco (1985). These authors, however, did not specify the period of time during which they observed the patients. Three master's-prepared nurses reviewed and revised the 66-item instrument, which was developed on the basis of a literature review and the NANDA list. Data were collected specific to a patient and not to the nurse's perception of Noncompliance in general. Seven items were found to rank high both in terms of importance and frequency: behavioral denial; verbal denial; direct observation; personal statement; does not feel susceptible; does not feel vulnerable; and does not believe in the efficacy of therapy.

Pokorny (1985) conducted a study to identify and validate DCs and critical DCs for the nursing diagnosis Knowledge Deficit using the Gordon and Sweeney (1979) nurse-validation model. A random sample of 120 patient charts was selected via a computer retrieval system based on the presence of Knowledge Deficit. These charts were reviewed and analyzed to identify and validate the diagnosis. Content validity of the tool was established by a panel of five experts, and test–retest reliability was established by the investigator, who reviewed 10 randomly selected charts twice using the same tool, 2 weeks apart. All kappas equaled one. A verbalized statement of inadequate knowledge ($n = 31$) was the most frequently identified characteristic, followed by verbalized inadequate understanding of information ($n = 16$), and verbalized inadequate recall of information ($n = 16$).

The following two diagnoses reflect health problems in the area of parent–infant relationship: Maternal Attachment and Parenting Alteration. Avant (1979) used five actual cases to test provisional criteria and to observe for additional provisional criteria for the nursing diagnosis Maternal Attachment. An observational tool developed by Klaus and Kennell (1976) was used. Fifteen primigravidas and their infants were observed for 20 minutes during their feeding sessions. Mothers were healthy women who had delivered vaginally full-term, healthy infants. Eleven infants were females and four were males, and their ages ranged from 12 hours to 4 days. Two of the infants were breastfed. There seems to be reasonable support for the provisional criteria in the data. Two of the highest frequencies occurred in visual contact (e.g., mother's eyes on baby and "en face"), three in touch (e.g., close contact touching infant with fingertips and palms, cradle), one in positive affect (e.g., mother's attention completely on infant), four in reciprocal interaction (e.g., light sleep, drowsy, bottle out, and encompassing), and one in vocalization (e.g., talking). However, one must point out that interaction may be different between females and males, between the age of 12 hours and 4 days, and between bottle-fed and breastfed. Studies with bigger sample sizes with consideration given to these factors in the design are needed to clarify potential confounding variables and strengthen the results.

Nicoletti, Reitz, and Gordon (1982) examined postpartum discharge referrals and prenatal referrals to identify critical DCs of actual and Potential Parenting Alterations. Critical DCs were defined as those that were present with 100% agreement. One hundred and fifty-one diagnoses were identified with 722 observations. Eighty percent were potential whereas 20% were actual diagnoses. Authors described good clustering process, but they were not able to identify critical DCs with 100% agreement. Authors reported that their data suggest subsets of the parenting category, such as Maternal Attachment Deficit and Physical Baby Care Skills Deficit. This study gave evidence that Parenting is at a higher level of abstraction in the classification scheme than Maternal Attachment. If this is the case, any attempt to identify critical DCs of Parenting Alterations would not yield clinically useful data. New diagnoses at the same level as Maternal Attachment need to be developed to address health problems in the parent–child relationship area.

The following five nursing diagnoses address the health problems that deal broadly with self-concept. In terms of the level of abstractness, Self-Esteem, Body Image, Identity Confusion, and Powerlessness are under the broader category of self-concept. However, research on each of these diagnoses, including Self-Concept, is discussed separately in this chapter in order to present new findings associated with each diagnosis.

Morris (1985) and Morris and Lackey (1986) reported a study in which the behavioral and emotional components of the psychological construct Self-Concept were validated as they were altered by the diagnosis of cancer. A structured interview and checklist of the behavioral and emotional components were used. Construct validity of the two instruments was determined by three oncology nurse experts. Thirty subjects who had been diagnosed as having cancer at least 3 months before (Group A) completed the checklist twice at 48-hour intervals. Another 30 subjects who had been diagnosed as having cancer for the first time completed the interview and the checklist between 6 and 8 weeks after diagnosis (Group B). Many patients (no numbers were specified by the authors) reported feeling hopeful, worthwhile, in control, calm, accepted, and loved; these results are in contrast to previously reported literature. Because of this, the investigators concluded that the behavioral and emotional components of self-concept were not altered by cancer as previously believed.

Using Fehring's CDV model methodology (1986), Norris and Kunes-Connell (1985, 1987) established the clinical validity of a nursing diagnosis, Disturbance in Self-Esteem. Two psychiatric CNSs assessed four groups of patients: (a) hospitalized psychiatric patients ($n = 10$); (b) chronically ill patients who were receiving home health care in the community ($n = 9$); (c) residents in a domestic abuse shelter ($n = 6$); and (d) adolescents in a chemical dependency treatment center and adult patients in chemical dependency treatment ($n = 31$). Those identified as having low self-esteem and who agreed to participate were included in the study. Defining characteristics with CDV score of >0.5 were: "lack of eye contact, self-negating verbalization, and evaluates self as unable to deal with situations."

Baird (1985) studied Altered Body Image in immobilized patients using a qualitative, descriptive methodology. A nursing body image assessment tool (Baird Body Image Assessment Tool, BBIAT) was developed and tested on 10 immobilized patients by five staff nurses and three expert nurses (two with associate degrees and one with a diploma in nursing). Patients were chosen from an orthopedic unit having a high number of patient referrals to a psychiatric clinical nurse specialist (CNS) concerning body image disturbance. Each patient was assessed three times in one day by three different nurses to test reliability and develop consensual validity. Following assessment by the staff and expert nurses, the investigator conducted an audiotaped interview with the same 10 patients using an equivalent assessment form and an unstructured interview schedule containing questions comparable to the BBIAT. Patients were assessed and interviewed by all three groups of nurses either on the day of surgery or the first postoperative day while prescribed bed rest was being maintained. Although the investigator took careful steps to develop the assessment tool on immobilized patients, questions included in the BBIAT were general and not focused on the aspect of immobility. Hence, the relationship between Altered Body Image and immobility remains unclear. Further, patients assessed for this study were too ill to evaluate body image. The author's reasoning for the selection of this time period was to meet the criteria of bed rest. Although this reason is reality based, the results may not be theoretically sound. The problem of body image may emerge over a longer period of time than was selected in this study. This author concurs with Baird that formal statistical analysis, with data from a bigger sample and expanded items, is needed to validate its use in practice.

Adolescent Identity Confusion was studied by Oldaker (1985). One hundred and thirty-eight adolescents (35% white males and 65% white females) responded to the Comrey Personality Scales (CPS) (Comrey, 1970) and the Psychiatric Epidemiological Research Interview (PERI) symptom scales (Dohrenwend, Shrout, Egri, & Mendelsohn, 1980); these were modified for adolescents. Four independent symptom dimensions emerged from the data and these were analyzed by principle axis factor analysis using varimax rotations. Any factor with a coefficient score of at least +0.40 was accepted as a component of a factor. Factored symptom clusters associated with anxiety, antisocial behavior, depression, and confusion were consistent with theory descriptors of Adolescent Identity Confusion. Authors proposed four nursing diagnoses related to developmental difficulties among adolescents: identity confusion related to problems of intimacy, negative identity, diffusion of time perspective, and diffusion of industry. Although the presentation of Erikson's (1968) constructs associated with each of these four nursing diagnoses is informative, these associations need clinical testing.

Miller (1984) developed and validated Powerlessness. The validation method included clinical observation/development of the definition of the nursing diagnosis and theoretical propositions and practice speculation through literature review, field observation, and refinement of critical indicators of the diagnosis. Field observation involved observations made at varying times during the day for 6 weeks using a participant observation method. To refine critical indicators, data were collected by 27 graduate students who made the nursing diagnosis of powerlessness on 81 chronically ill patients using the Impact of Chronic Illness Inventory (Miller, 1980). Sixteen categories of the indicators were found; these were classified by a panel of 24 experts as severe, moderate, low, or no powerlessness. Those characteristics in the severe category were labeled critical indicators. However, equating the severe category with critical indicators is troublesome because indicators in other categories can be critical but of lesser severity.

In general, research on the area of self-concept needs to be further delineated in order to make each nursing diagnosis clinically more sensitive and specific for its use. The efforts undertaken by these investigators represent a beginning phase of research development.

CONCLUSIONS AND FUTURE DIRECTIONS

Since the publication of the Gordons review (1985), the growth of nursing diagnosis research, both in quantity and quality, is remarkable. Numerous research methodologies proposed have been found to be useful by several investigators. Critical examination of validation studies revealed considerable evidence of investigator's acute awareness of and careful attention to validity and reliability issues of tools. That many investigators have utilized clinical experts in their validation efforts is meritorious. However, the qualification of experts is of concern since it varied from nurses with associate degrees and diplomas to master's and doctoral preparation. Given the same clinical experience, nurses with advanced degrees should be considered experts; their expertise can be regarded as the yardstick for measuring clinical judgment and decision making.

It is regrettable that a majority of investigators failed to address the external validity of their results. Hence, most studies do not provide conclusive data for generalization. The majority of studies need to be replicated with larger sample sizes, different patient populations, and randomized national samples. Likewise, numerous investigations suffered from limitations such as being pilot in nature, using convenience samples, and having a one-group design.

Therefore, the challenge for research on nursing diagnosis remains strong as investigators strive to identify new methodologies for refinement and validation of new nursing diagnoses. Definition of nursing diagnoses and etiologies as well as criterion measures for defining characteristics are some of the basic elements that are yet to be refined. Development and validation of nursing diagnoses for aggregates (i.e., community nursing diagnoses) is one area of study that will require a concerted effort by community nurse experts. Likewise, testing conceptual frameworks for a nursing diagnosis taxonomy is another area of research that warrants careful attention.

Research on nursing diagnosis is the key to the success of nursing diagnoses. Further development of valid and reliable nursing diagnoses will contribute to the advancement of nursing practice and knowledge development of nursing science.

REFERENCES

American Nurses' Association. (1980). *Nursing: A social policy statement.* Kansas City, MO: Author.

Avant, K. (1979). Nursing diagnosis: Maternal attachment. *Advances in Nursing Science, 2*(1), 45–55.

Baas, L. S., & Allen, G. A. (1985). Memory error: Developing a new nursing diagnosis. *Nursing Clinics of North America, 70,* 731–743.

Baird, S. (1985). Development of a nursing assessment tool to diagnose altered body image in immobilized patients. *Orthopedic Nursing, 4*(1), 47–54.

Baldwin, K. A., & Lueckenotte, A. G. (1986). Use of nursing diagnoses in community health agencies using the PORS. In M. E. Hurley (Ed.), *Classification of nursing diagnosis: Proceedings of the sixth conference North American Nursing Diagnosis Association* (pp. 330–337). St. Louis, MO: Mosby.

Burke, L. J., Gabriel, L. M., Fischer, L. E., & Zemke, S. L. (1986). Nursing diagnosis, indicators, and interventions in an outpatient cardiac rehabilitation program. *Heart & Lung, 15,* 70–76.

Castle, M. R. (1982). Interrater agreement in the use of nursing diagnosis. In M. J. Kim & D. A. Moritz (Eds.), *Classification of nursing diagnoses: Proceedings of the Third and Fourth National Conferences* (pp. 153–167). New York: McGraw-Hill.

Cattaneo, C. J., & Lackey, N. R. (1987). Impaired skin integrity. In A. M. McLane (Ed.), *Classification of nursing diagnoses: Proceedings of the seventh conference North American Nursing Diagnosis Association* (pp. 129-135). St. Louis, MO: Mosby.

Comrey, A. L. (1970). *EDITS Manual: Comrey Personality Scales.* San Diego, CA: EDITS Publishers.

Creason, N. S., Pogue, N. J., Nelson, A. A., & Hoyt, C. A. (1985). Validating the nursing diagnosis of impaired physical mobility. *Nursing Clinics of North America, 20,* 669-683.

Dalton, J. (1985). A descriptive study: Defining characteristics of the nursing diagnosis cardiac output, alterations in: decreased. *Image: The Journal of Nursing Scholarship, 17,* 113-117.

Dohrenwend, B. F., Shrout, P. E., Egri, G., & Mendelsohn, F. S. (1980). Nonspecific psychological distress and other dimensions of psychopathology. *Archives of General Psychiatry, 37,* 1229-1236.

Dougherty, C. (1985). The nursing diagnosis of decreased cardiac output. *Nursing Clinics of North America, 20,* 787-799.

Erikson, E. H. (1968). *Identity youth and crisis.* New York: Norton.

Fadden, T., Fehring, R. J., & Kenkel-Rossi, E. (1987). Validation studies: Paper presentations. In A. M. McLane (Ed.), *Classification of nursing diagnoses: Proceedings of the sixth conference North American Nursing Diagnosis Association* (pp. 113-120). St. Louis, MO: Mosby.

Fehring, R. J. (1986). Validation. In M. E. Hurley (Ed.), *Classification of nursing diagnoses: Proceedings of the sixth conference North American Nursing Diagnosis Association* (pp. 183-190). St. Louis, MO: Mosby.

Frenn, M. D., Jacobs, C. A., Lee, H. A., Sanger, M. T., & Strong, K. A. (1987). Delphi survey to gain consensus on wellness and health promotion nursing diagnoses. In A. M. McLane (Ed.), *Classification of nursing diagnoses: Proceedings of the seventh conference North American Nursing Diagnosis Association* (pp. 154-159). St. Louis, Mo: Mosby.

Gebbie, K. M. (1976). Research project. In K. M. Gebbie (Ed.), *Summary of the second national conference classification of nursing diagnoses* (pp. 19-21). St. Louis, MO: Clearinghouse, National Group for Classification of Nursing Diagnoses.

Gebbie, K. M., & Lavin, M. A. (Eds.). (1975). *Proceedings of the first national conference classification of nursing diagnoses.* St. Louis, MO: Mosby.

Gordon, M. (1982). *Nursing diagnosis: Process and application.* New York: McGraw-Hill.

Gordon, M. (1985). Nursing diagnosis. In H. H. Werley & J. J. Fitzpatrick (Eds.), *Annual Review of Nursing Research.* New York: Springer Publishing Co.

Gordon, M., & Sweeney, M. A. (1979). Methodological problems and issues in identifying and standardizing nursing diagnosis. *Advances in Nursing Science, 2*(1), 1-15.

Gould, M. T. (1983). Nursing diagnoses concurrent with multiple sclerosis. *Journal of Neurosurgical Nursing, 15,* 339-345.

Guzzetta, C. E., & Forsyth, G. L. (1979). Nursing diagnostic pilot study: Psychophysiologic stress. *Advances in Nursing Science, 2*(1), 27-44.

Hartley, W. S. (1970). *Manual for the twenty-statements problem (whom am I).* Kansas City, KS: Department of Human Ecology and Community Health, University of Kansas Medical Center.

Hoskins, L. M., McFarlane, E. A., Rubenfeld, M. G., Walsh, M. B., & Schreier, A. M. (1986). Nursing diagnosis in the chronically ill: Methodology for clinical validation. *Advances in Nursing Science, 8*(3), 80–89.

Hubalik, K., & Kim, M. J. (1984). Nursing diagnoses associated with heart failure in critical care nursing. In M. J. Kim, G. K. McFarland, & A. M. McLane (Eds.), *Classification of nursing diagnoses: Proceedings of the fifth national conference* (pp. 139–149). St. Louis, MO: Mosby.

Hurley, M. E. (Ed.). (1986). *Classification of nursing diagnoses: Proceedings of the sixth conference North American Nursing Diagnosis Association.* St. Louis, MO: Mosby.

Janken, J. K., & Reynolds, B. A. (1987). Identifying patients with the potential for falling. In A. M. McLane (Ed.), *Classification of nursing diagnoses: Proceedings of the seventh conference North American Nursing Diagnosis Association* (pp. 136–143). St. Louis, MO: Mosby.

Jones, P. E. (1982a). Developing terminology: A University of Toronto experience. In M. J. Kim & D. A. Moritz (Eds.), *Classification of nursing diagnoses: Proceedings of the third and fourth national conferences* (pp. 138–145). New York: McGraw-Hill.

Jones, P. E. (1982b). The revision of nursing diagnosis terms (1980). In M. J. Kim & D. A. Moritz (Eds.), *Classification of nursing diagnoses: Proceedings of the third and fourth national conferences* (pp. 196–203). New York: McGraw-Hill.

Kerlinger, F. N. (1973). *Foundations of behavioral research,* 2nd ed. New York: Holt, Rinehart and Winston.

Kim, M. J., Amoroso, R., Gulanick, M., Moyer, K., Parsons, E., Scherubel, J., Stafford, M., Suhayda, R., & Yocum, C. (1982). Clinical use of nursing diagnoses in cardiovascular nursing. In M. J. Kim & D. A. Moritz (Eds.), *Classification of nursing diagnoses: Proceedings of the third and fourth national conferences* (pp. 184–190). New York: McGraw-Hill.

Kim, M. J., Amoroso-Seritella, R., Gulanick, M., Moyer, K., Parsons, E., Scherubel, J., Stafford, M., Suhayda, R., & Yocum, C. (1984). Clinical validation of cardiovascular nursing diagnoses. In M. J. Kim, G. K. McFarland, & A. M. McLane (Eds.), *Classification of nursing diagnoses: Proceedings of the fifth national conference* (pp. 128–137). St. Louis, MO: Mosby.

Kim, M. J., McFarland, G. K., & McLane, A. M. (1984). *Classification of nursing diagnoses: Proceedings of the fifth national conference.* St. Louis, MO: Mosby.

Kim, M. J., & Moritz, D. A. (Eds.). (1982). *Classification of nursing diagnoses: Proceedings of the third and fourth national conferences.* New York: McGraw-Hill.

Klaus, M., & Kennell, J. (1976). *Maternal infant bonding.* St. Louis, MO: Mosby.

Lackey, N. R. (1986). Use of the Q methodology in validating defining characteristics of special nursing diagnoses. In M. E. Hurley (Ed.), *Classification of nursing diagnoses: Proceedings of the sixth conference North American Nursing Diagnosis Association* (pp. 191–196). St. Louis, MO: Mosby.

Lawson, K., & Lackey, N. R. (1986). Development of an instrument to measure altered levels of awareness in significant others who have experienced psychological impact. In M. E. Hurley (Ed.), *Classification of nursing diagnoses: Proceedings of the sixth conference North American Nursing Diagnosis Association* (pp. 349–359). St. Louis, MO: Mosby.

Lo, C. K., & Kim, M. J. (1986). Construct validity of sleep pattern disturbance: A methodological approach. In M. E. Hurley (Ed.), *Classification of nursing diagnoses: Proceedings of the sixth conference North American Nursing Diagnosis Association* (pp. 197–206). St. Louis, MO: Mosby.

Martin, K. S. (1982). Community health research in nursing diagnosis: The Omaha study. In M. J. Kim & D. A. Moritz (Eds.), *Classification of nursing diagnoses: Proceedings of the third and fourth national conferences* (pp. 167–175). New York: McGraw-Hill.

McFarland, G. K., & Naschinski, C. (1985). Impaired communication. *Nursing Clinics of North America, 20,* 775–785.

McKeehan, K. M., & Gordon, M. (1982). Utilization of accepted nursing diagnoses. In M. J. Kim & D. A. Moritz (Eds.), *Classification of nursing diagnoses: Proceedings of the third and fourth national conferences* (pp. 190–195). New York: McGraw-Hill.

McLane, A. M. (Ed.). (1987). *Classification of nursing diagnoses: Proceedings of the seventh conference North American Nursing Diagnosis Association.* St. Louis, MO: Mosby.

McShane, R. E., & McLane, A. M. (1985). Constipation: Consensual and empirical validation. *Nursing Clinics of North America, 20,* 801–808.

Metzger, K. L., & Hiltunen, E. F. (1987). Diagnostic content validation of ten frequently reported nursing diagnoses. In A. M. McLane (Ed.), *Classification of nursing diagnoses: Proceedings of the seventh conference North American Nursing Diagnosis Association* (pp. 144–153). St. Louis, MO: Mosby.

Miller, J. F. (1980). A practitioner/teacher role for graduate program faculty. In L. Machan (Ed.), *The practitioner teacher role: Practice what you teach.* Wakefield, MA: Nursing Resources.

Miller, J. F. (1984). Development and validation of a diagnostic label: Powerlessness. In M. J. Kim, G. K. McFarland, & A. M. McLane (Eds.), *Classification of nursing diagnoses: Proceedings of the fifth national conference* (pp. 116–127). St. Louis, MO: Mosby.

Morris, C. A. (1985). Self-concept as altered by the diagnoses of cancer. *Nursing Clinics of North America, 20,* 611–630.

Morris, C. A., & Lackey, N. R. (1986). A description of self-concept as it is altered by the diagnoses of cancer. In M. E. Hurley (Ed.), *Classification of nursing diagnoses: Proceedings of the sixth conference North American Nursing Diagnosis Association* (pp. 370–379). St. Louis, MO: Mosby.

Munns, D. C. (1985). A validation of the defining characteristics of the nursing diagnosis "Potential for Violence." *Nursing Clinics of North America, 20,* 711–722.

Nicoletti, A. M., Reitz, S. E., & Gordon, M. (1982). A descriptive study of the parenting diagnosis (1980). In M. J. Kim & D. A. Moritz (Eds.), *Classification of nursing diagnoses: Proceedings of the third and fourth national conferences* (pp. 176–183). New York: McGraw-Hill.

Norris, J., & Kunes-Connell, M. (1985). Self-esteem disturbance. *Nursing Clinics of North America, 20,* 745–761.

Norris, J., & Kunes-Connell, M. (1987). Self-esteem disturbance: A clinical validation study. In A. M. McLane (Ed.), *Classification of nursing* diagnoses: Proceedings of the seventh conference North American Nursing Diagnosis Association (pp. 121–128). St. Louis, MO: Mosby.

Oldaker, S. M. (1985). Identity confusion: A nursing diagnosis for adolescents. Nursing Clinics of North America, 20, 763–773.

Pokorny, B. (1985). Validating a diagnostic label: Knowledge deficits. Nursing Clinics of North America, 20, 641–655.

Ryan, P., & Falco, S. M. (1985). A pilot study to validate the defining characteristics of the nursing diagnosis of noncompliance. Nursing Clinics of North America, 20, 685–695.

Sgroi, S. M., Holland, J. C. B., & Solkoff, N. (1970). Development of an anxiety-depression scale for use with medically ill patients. Mimeograph. Department of Psychiatry, School of Medicine, State University of New York at Buffalo.

Shoemaker, J. K. (1984). Essential features of a nursing diagnosis. In M. J. Kim, G. K. McFarland, & A. M. McLane (Eds.), Classification of nursing diagnoses: Proceedings of the fifth national conference (pp. 104–112). St. Louis, MO: Mosby.

Silver, S. M., Halfmann, T. M., McShane, R. E., Hunt, C. A., & Nowak, C. A. (1984). The identification of clinically recorded nursing diagnoses and indicators. In M. J. Kim, G. K. McFarland, & A. M. McLane (Eds.), Classification of nursing diagnoses: Proceedings of the fifth national conference (pp. 162–165). St. Louis, MO: Mosby.

Spielberger, C. D., Gorsuch, R. L., and Lushene, R. E. (1970). Manual for the State-Trait Anxiety Inventory. Palo Alto, CA: Consulting Psychologist Press.

Suhayda, R., & Kim, M. J. (1984). Documentation of nursing process in critical care. In M. J. Kim, G. K. McFarland, & A. M. McLane (Eds.), Classification of nursing diagnoses: Proceedings of the fifth national conference (pp. 166–172). St. Louis, MO: Mosby.

Vincent, K. G. (1985a). The validation of a nursing diagnosis. Nursing Clinics of North America, 20, 631–640.

Vincent, K. G. (1985b). The validation of a nursing diagnosis: Nurse-consensus survey. In M. E. Hurley (Ed.), Classification of nursing diagnoses: Proceedings of the sixth conference North American Nursing Diagnosis Association (pp. 207–214). St. Louis, MO: Mosby.

Voith, A. M., & Smith, D. A. (1985). Validation of the nursing diagnoses of urinary retention. Nursing Clinics of North America, 20, 723–729.

Wessel, S. L., & Kim, M. J. (1984). Nursing functions related to the nursing diagnosis decreased cardiac output. In M. J. Kim, G. K. McFarland, & A. M. McLane (Eds.), Classification of nursing diagnoses: Proceedings of the fifth national conference (pp. 192–198). St. Louis, MO: Mosby.

York, K. (1985). Clinical validation of two respiratory nursing diagnoses and their defining characteristics. Nursing Clinics of North America, 20, 657–667.

Chapter 7

Patient Contracting

SUSAN BOEHM
SCHOOL OF NURSING
THE UNIVERSITY OF MICHIGAN

CONTENTS

The purpose of this review was to examine the research on patient contracting that has appeared in the nursing literature since the early 1970s. During the past 15 years, well over 300 research articles on this topic have been published in the nonnursing literature, compared to approximately 20 articles in the nursing literature. Fewer than eight of the nursing articles were identified as research-based. A comprehensive survey of works that were published by nurses from 1965 to 1986 was undertaken for this review. Titles, abstracts, and articles that referred to contracts were identified by computer and manual searches of the literature in nursing and related fields. Published and unpublished theses, dissertations, and reports were sought. Each of the identified research-based articles is included to identify strengths and weaknesses and to stimulate higher-quality research in the future.

Research on patient contracting within nursing is in the early developmental stages. The paucity of research and the number of studies using descriptive and preexperimental designs reflect this fact. Thus, for this review, studies were included that were descriptive as well as those in which true or quasi-experimental designs were used.

A major limitation of the review was the inability to identify nurses who published in other than nursing journals. Although an extensive list of personal contacts was used for this purpose and attempts were made to confirm the author as a nurse, appropriate authors still may have been excluded.

The chapter begins with a brief overview of patient contracting and a discussion of the major conceptual issues and problems. Because it is apparent that patient contracting only recently has generated interest among nurses, several of the articles include preliminary work that is intended as a foundation for further study. Such studies serve an important function in that they point to areas that require further clarification of operational definitions and, most importantly, clarification of the underlying principles guiding the contracting process.

BACKGROUND OF PATIENT CONTRACTING

Contract negotiation with patients and clients developed predominately in a behavioral framework with the intention of actively involving clients in their treatment. The majority of the research literature on contracting is found in the journals of psychology and social work beginning in the early 1970s. More recently it has been indexed under such headings as behavioral medicine and patient compliance.

Contingency Contracts

By far, the approach and form of the patient contract most frequently reported is that of the contingency contract. Contingency contracts, used as a means of learning and changing behavior, evolved from the early behavior modification treatment programs and have continued to be developed within the growing field of behavior analysis and behavioral health and medicine. Consequently, contracting has been applied and tested in wide and diverse settings.

The contingency contract is based upon the principle of positive reinforcement. Researchers who have studied this principle have demonstrated a relationship between behavior and environment. The principle of positive reinforcement is based on the assumption that a desired behavior can be increased by providing reinforcement for that behavior (Ayllon & Azrin, 1968). Thus, the provision of favorable consequences for the performance of specified behaviors increases the probability that the patient will repeat the reinforced behavior; this reinforcement may be used to increase learning, adherence, or self-care. The contingency contract is a technique in which the desired behaviors are specified clearly and favorable consequences are identified in advance; thus appropriate rewards can be provided when the behavior has been performed successfully.

Therefore, contingency contracting is defined as the systematic arrangement for the reception of a reward in return for performance of a specific behavior (Kazdin, 1975). A written contract is signed by both parties, which contains specifications of both the behavior to be performed and the desired reinforcer.

Evidence is beginning to emerge that demonstrates the application of principles of positive reinforcement in nursing practice. In their now classic article, Ayllon and Michael (1959) were the first to describe the effectiveness of nurses using reinforcement principles in a mental health facility. More recently, a review of the use of techniques of positive reinforcement in nursing was published by Lebow (1973). Specific examples include use of positive reinforcement in the control of chronic pain (Fowler, Fordyce, & Berni, 1969) and the rehabilitation of patients with spinal cord injuries (Rottkamp, 1976).

Treatment Contracts

Whereas the use of the contingency contract is the type of contract most widely reported in the research literature over the past 15 years, the treatment contract also has been reported (Rosen, 1978). The treatment contract is structured in a legalistic manner and is an attempt to formalize the planning of treatment programs. Such a contract includes the treatment goals, a time limit, the treatment methods and personnel involved, and the degree and type of patient involvement. Finally, the contract is signed by the patient and personnel.

The contingency contract and the treatment contract are very different. The former is based on the principles of environmental contingencies, whereas the latter is founded on the therapeutic work to be accomplished between the client and therapist (Rosen, 1978). The underlying assumption of the treatment contract is that the therapist and client agree that the therapist will provide skills and time to the patient. In return, the patient will present the problem openly and honestly, submit to the therapist's expertise, and pay for the services (Rosen, 1978).

REVIEW OF RESEARCH

Contingency Contracts

The earliest descriptions of the contingency contract in the nursing literature appeared in the 1970s. Steckel (1974) used reinforcement contracts written with patients on dialysis for the control of potassium levels in an exploratory case study, and also in a study (Steckel, 1976b) where contracts were written with staff nurses (rather than patients) to increase the nursing assessment.

The purpose of the study by Deimling et al. (1984) was to test the effectiveness of patient education and contingency contracting with patients who were on dialysis and seeking to achieve better phosphorus control. The patients were assigned randomly to one of three groups, consisting of a control group and two experimental groups. The first experimental group received an educational intervention, and the second received the educational intervention with contingency contracting. Although the data indicated a statistically significant increase in knowledge scores for all three groups, the largest difference was seen in the contracting group. There were no differences in the phosphorus levels between the groups.

The authors discussed the limitations of the study that might have accounted for the lack of significant differences. Additionally, however, there were major methodological flaws in the study. The authors hypothesized that patients who received contingency contracting combined with an educational intervention would demonstrate better phosphorus control than patients in the other groups. They did not define contingency, however, and there was no mention of contingencies in the definition of contracting. To be more specific, because the definition of contracting did not include contingencies, the contract that was implemented was essentially a treatment contract. There was no indication that patients received contingencies for the completion of the contract. Apparently the authors did not distinguish contingency contracts sufficiently from other types of contracts in planning the study. Furthermore, it was difficult to evaluate the process and effectiveness of the contracting because the behaviors for which the patients contracted were not discussed. The behaviors were referred to as mutually agreed upon goals related to the control of phosphorus levels. It was not clear whether these behaviors were broken down systematically into small steps so as to shape new behavior, according to reinforcement theory, or whether the goals were chosen according to the principles of goal setting. From the discussion of the phosphate control algorithm that was used for implementing the physician's standing orders, one could assume that steps in the algorithm were the focus for patients' behaviors in the contract; however, the behaviors should have been stated explicitly.

Van Dover (1986) evaluated the effectiveness of two types of contracts written with sexually active college women in an effort to prevent unplanned pregnancies. One group of subjects negotiated contracts without reinforcement, and one group negotiated contracts for a reinforcer received in return for performance of an identified behavior. Thus, the design of the study provided the opportunity to compare the effectiveness of the treatment contract with the contingency contract.

The design for the study (Van Dover, 1986) was a pretest/posttest field experiment. The sample included 152 sexually active female outpatients, ages 18 to 22 years, from the student gynecology clinic of a large university. Subjects were selected randomly and assigned randomly to one of three groups. The control group received routine clinic care, and a second group received routine clinic care, an educational component, and contracting without reinforcement. The third group received routine clinic care, education, and contracting with patient-chosen reinforcers that were received when the contract was met.

Findings revealed a significant increase in knowledge and consistency in use of contraception for both contracting groups. However, since both experimental groups also received an educational component, the educational and contracting effects were confounded. In addition, subjects who received reinforcers fulfilled more contracts, were more likely to say that the process of contracting was valuable to them, were more likely to discuss their contracts with others, and were more likely to discuss birth control with their sex partners. Those subjects who did not receive reinforcement were more likely than the reinforcement group or control group to leave the study before the treatment was complete.

The use of contingency contracts also has been studied in an attempt to improve patient education and patient compliance among hypertensive patients in a series of three studies using a cohort design (Steckel, 1976a; Steckel & Swain, 1977; Swain & Steckel, 1981). Outpatients from hypertension clinics were selected and assigned randomly to one of three groups: routine care, patient education, and contingency contracting. In these studies, those who wrote contracts with reinforcers demonstrated significantly better knowledge scores on the posttest, kept more clinic appointments, and had decreased diastolic blood pressure. However, a weakness of all three studies was that the contracts were negotiated with the patients by one clinical nurse specialist, thus creating the possibility of a positive interaction effect between the nurse and patients.

The effectiveness of contingency contracting was investigated further with patients who had a chronic illness, specifically, arthritis, diabetes, or hypertension (Steckel & Funnell, 1981). The patients in two major hospital outpatient departments were assigned randomly to the nursing staff normally employed in the settings. Each nurse contracted with patients who had one of the three chronic illnesses; outcomes were assessed for different diagnoses using subgroups. Patients who negotiated contracts for adherence to an aspect of their prescribed medical regimen demonstrated significantly better results relative to appointment keeping, weight loss, and blood pressure reduction than those in the control group. There were no differences between groups in the fasting blood sugar levels of the patients with diabetes. In addition, a variety of psychosocial tests were given to the subjects every 6 months. Those who negotiated contracts tended to perceive themselves as healthier and more capable of managing their illness than the comparison group.

Treatment Contracts

The development of treatment contracts in nursing can be seen in the preliminary work by Loomis (1982, 1985). It is important to note that the differences between Loomis's treatment contract and the contingency contract are not limited to the absence of reinforcing contingencies. The most significant difference is that transactional analysis provided the conceptual framework for Loomis's treatment contract as compared to the conceptual framework of reinforcement theory in the contingency contract. Consequently, the rationale, the format, and the process of negotiating the contracts differ because of the different principles that are involved.

Variations of treatment contracts were seen in the nursing literature. Langford (1978) described a contract that was built on the nursing process. Hayes and Davis (1980) described the use of the health care contract in a primary care setting. In addition, behavioral treatment contracts were used with patients who had borderline personality disorders (McEnany & Tescher, 1985), as an intervention for the obese patient (White, 1986), and to increase compliance for patients with black lung disease (Thomson & Willis, 1982).

In another example of the treatment contract, Herje (1980) described a contract that involves the patient in goal setting and states that "the goals are stated in measurable behaviors, (small, achievable goals have a greater chance of success)" (Herje, 1980, p. 30). However, this description of the contract was confusing because of the inclusion of two different sets of principles. Specifically, Herje emphasized both goal setting, an element of treatment contracting, and reinforcing consequences of a successful outcome, an element of contingency contracting. Ultimately, the successful testing of the usefulness of contracting requires clear distinction of the principles and conceptual framework to be followed.

Helgeson and Berg (1985) conducted a descriptive pilot study focused on the development and implementation of treatment contracts. The contract described by the authors incorporated concepts of the treatment contract as well as concepts of quality assurance. The contracts were implemented by senior nursing students in their community health nursing course. The format, developed by the authors, included the client's view of his/her needs and goals, as well as the needs and goals identified by the nurse. The mutually agreed upon needs and problems were identified and prioritized, and objectives and process outcomes were specified for use in evaluation. The authors identified two phases of the project: the development and implementation of the contracting process, and an evaluation of the reactions of the students and clients to the process of contracting.

Although the authors discussed the contracting process relative to each of four home visits, the underlying principles that provided the link between the contracts and the quality assurance program were not stated clearly. The intent appears to be that quality assurance could be facilitated as a result of the explicitness of the contract. However, the relationship between contracting and quality assurance was developed inadequately. Also, there was a lack of clarity because of the absence of defined concepts and principles that would have provided the framework and guided the implementation of contracting. Goal setting was discussed broadly, but it was never specified as the conceptual framework. The lack of a specific framework was confused further by the equal emphasis that was given to a review of the contingency contracting literature.

The second phase of the study involved the use of a questionnaire that was given to the clients and students in order to evaluate their reactions to the use of the contracts. A convenience sample was used, and the authors pointed out that the sample size was inadequate for statistical analysis. A discussion of the responses to the questionnaire indicated favorable reactions to the use of the contracting process by both students and clients.

SUMMARY AND IMPLICATIONS FOR FUTURE RESEARCH

It is difficult to draw conclusions about either treatment or contingency contracts because of the paucity of nursing research reported to date. However, based on the contracting research in related disciplines and upon the few studies of contracting in nursing, it appears to be an area worthy of further exploration. There are characteristics of patient contracting that complement and build upon the nurse–patient relationship. The theoretical frameworks such as reinforcement theory, transactional analysis, and goal setting have a potential for enhancing the effectiveness of the work the nurse and patient carry out together. In addition, the process of contracting may specify and illuminate nursing's unique contribution.

The quality and rigor of the work reported here covered a wide range. The lack of well-developed problem statements and operational definitions for the studies was apparent. In addition, the confusion about or lack of theoretical framework on which to base the contract needs to be rectified in future studies. In one study, the lack of clarity about the underlying principles resulted in a contract built on the principles of goal setting in the same manner as one would build on the principles of shaping a new behavior. The underlying principles that govern the process are very different for goal setting compared to shaping new behaviors. Future research will be more useful when increased attention is given to the operational definitions as well as to the underlying theoretical framework.

This lack of attention to the details of the contract and the process of negotiating the contract require careful deliberation and description in future studies. For example, whether the behaviors are chosen by the nurse, a medical protocol, or the patient needs to be identified. In addition, how the reinforcer is negotiated, when the reinforcer will be delivered, and how the behavior is measured to indicate the reception of the reinforcer requires description.

In some cases the research design and the sampling techniques were not described adequately. In other instances the contracting was implemented as a part of a more elaborate treatment program, and it was not possible to account for the effectiveness of the contracting.

Although the behavioral strategy of patient contracting was found most frequently in the literature dealing with patient compliance, a potential for the use of contracting also lies within the realm of encouraging a patient to achieve behavior change. There is opportunity for a patient to implement the contracting process as a means of managing a chronic illness rather than simply to comply with medical regimens. Indeed, a major potential for future studies is to perceive the patient as the pivotal person capable of negotiating contracts not only with the nurse, but also with other individuals in the environment who will, in turn, support the patient's new and desired behaviors. Behaviors to be supported include those involved in health maintenance, as well as the management of illness.

Generally, the literature tends to point to the use of contracting in long-term chronic illnesses. However, the short-term use of such contracts in an acute-care setting has not been explored. For example, weaning the patient from a ventilator, implementing postoperative deep-breathing and coughing, and self-care of wounds and dressings appear to be areas with potential patient response to reinforcement as implemented in the contracting process.

Perhaps contracting to improve management of health and illness may be learned better as a young adult or even as a child. The principles and techniques involved have been used effectively in educational and mental health settings with younger age groups. Thus, teaching the younger individual these techniques in order to maintain health, prevent accidents, and manage illness may result in habits that will be particularly useful in preventing disease and managing illness during the adult life.

Finally, although nurses generally are familiar with behavioral interventions such as contracting, few are prepared to analyze their own behaviors from a perspective that they as nurses provide contingencies that shape patients' behaviors. In other words, future research is needed to provide behavioral analysis of the complex contingencies that nurses unintentionally provide that influence patient behavior.

REFERENCES

Ayllon, T., & Azrin, N. H. (1968). *The token economy.* New York: Appleton-Century-Crofts.

Ayllon, T., & Michael, J. (1959). The psychiatric nurse as a behavioral engineer. *Journal of the Experimental Analysis of Behavior, 2,* 323–324.

Deimling, A., Denny, M., Harrison, M., Kerr, B., Mayfield, B., Pelle-Shearer, M., Seaby, N., & Townsend, S. (1984). Effect of an algorithm and patient information on serum phosphorus levels. *American Nephrology Nurses' Association Journal, 11*(1), 35–39, 50.

Fowler, R. S., Fordyce, W. E., & Berni, R. (1969). Operant conditioning in chronic illness. *American Journal of Nursing, 69,* 1226–1228.

Hayes, W. S., & Davis, L. L. (1980). What is a health care contract? *Health Values, 4*(2), 82–86, 89.

Helgeson, D. M., & Berg, C. L. (1985). A method of health promotion. *Journal of Community Health Nursing, 2,* 199–207.

Herje, P. A. (1980). Hows and whys of patient contracting. *Nurse Educator, 5*(1), 30–34.

Kazdin, A. E. (1975). *Behavior modification in applied settings.* Homewood, IL: The Dorsey Press.

Langford, T. (1978). Establishing a nursing contract. *Nursing Outlook, 26,* 386–388.

Lebow, M. (1973). *A significant method in nursing practice.* Englewood Cliffs, NJ: Prentice-Hall.

Loomis, M. (1982). Contracting for change. *Transactional Analysis Journal, 12*(1), 51–55.

Loomis, M. (1985). Levels of contracting. *Journal of Psychosocial Nursing, 23*(3), 9–14.

McEnany, G. W., & Tescher, B. E. (1985). Contracting for care: One nursing approach to the hospitalized borderline patient. *Journal of Psychosocial Nursing, 23*(4), 11–18.

Rosen, B. (1978). Written treatment contracts: Their use in planning treatment programs for inpatients. *British Journal of Psychiatry, 133,* 410–415.

Rottkamp, B. S. (1976). A behavior modification approach to nursing therapeutics in body positioning of spinal cord-injured patients. *Nursing Research, 25,* 181–186.

Steckel, S. B. (1974). The use of positive reinforcement in order to increase patient compliance. *American Association of Nephrology Nurses and Technicians Journal, 1*(1), 39–41.

Steckel, S. B. (1976a). Influence of knowledge and of contingency contracting on adherence to hypertensive treatment regimens. *Dissertation Abstracts International, 37,* 1180B. (University Microfilms No. 7619249)

Steckel, S. B. (1976b). Utilization of reinforcement contracts to increase written evidence of the nursing assessment. *Nursing Research, 25,* 58–61.

Steckel, S. B. (1980). Contracting with patient-selected reinforcers. *American Journal of Nursing, 80,* 1596–1599.

Steckel, S. B. (1982). Predicting, measuring, implementing and following up on patient compliance. *Nursing Clinics of North America, 17,* 491–498.

Steckel, S. B., & Funnell, M. M. (1981). *Increasing adherence of outpatients to therapeutic regimens.* Final Report on Veterans Administration Health Service Research and Development Project, #343. Ann Arbor, MI.

Steckel, S. B., & Swain, M. A. (1977). Contracting with patients to improve compliance. *Hospitals, 51,* 81–84.

Swain, M. A., & Steckel, S. B. (1981). Influencing adherence among hypertensives. *Research in Nursing and Health, 4,* 213–233.

Thomson, P. S., & Willis, J. C. (1982). Compliance challenges in a black lung clinic. *Nursing Clinics of North America, 17,* 513–521.

Van Dover, L. (1986a). Influence of nurse–client contracting on family planning knowledge and behaviors in a university student population. *Dissertation Abstracts International, 46,* 3787B. Unpublished doctoral dissertation, The University of Michigan, Ann Arbor, Michigan. (University Microfilms No. DA8600566).

White, J. H. (1986). Behavioral intervention for the obese client. *Nurse Practitioner, 11*(1), 27–28, 30, 32.

PART III

Research on Nursing Education

Chapter 8

Parent–Child Nursing Education

CHERYL S. ALEXANDER
JOHNS HOPKINS SCHOOL OF HYGIENE AND PUBLIC HEALTH

KARIN E. JOHNSON
SCHOOL OF NURSING AND HEALTH SCIENCES
SALISBURY STATE COLLEGE

CONTENTS

This review of research related to parent–child nursing education was compiled from studies published since 1970. During this period, many nursing curricula were expanded from a medical model focus on obstetrics and pediatrics to a more integrative focus on maternal and child nursing, parent–child nursing, and nursing of the childbearing and child-rearing family, or to a totally integrated curricular model. Paralleling the curricular changes were changes in the methods used to teach parent–child nursing content and changes in the format of state board examinations. In spite of the substantive nature of these changes, this review revealed a surprising paucity of research assessing their impact.

157

Studies included in this review were obtained from a computer search of nursing literature under a number of parent–child-nursing-related topics as well as topics related to nursing education. In addition, nursing indexes for each year were reviewed individually. The following topical areas were among those explored: parenting, school health, family nursing, women's health, child health, perinatal nursing, adolescence, obstetrical nursing, maternal and child health nursing, pediatric nursing, baccalaureate nursing education, graduate nursing education, associate degree nursing education, diploma nursing education, nursing curricula, specialization, and competency. Specific journal indexes including *Nursing Research, Nursing Outlook, Research in Nursing and Health, Journal of Nursing Education, Nursing and Health Care,* and *Maternal–Child Nursing* also were reviewed.

Literature presented in this review is divided into two sections: (a) literature related to undergraduate and graduate nursing curricula, and (b) literature related to prediction of success on state board examinations or in graduate school. In a final section the findings are summarized and suggestions for further research are proposed.

PARENT–CHILD NURSING CURRICULA

Issues related to parent–child nursing curricula at the undergraduate and graduate levels were explored either directly or indirectly in only seven studies. Baccalaureate curricular issues were addressed in four studies, and master's-level curricular issues in three studies. All of the studies were descriptive.

Baccalaureate Nursing Curricula

With the emergence of integrated baccalaureate nursing programs in the 1970s, research attention was centered on the impact of curricular changes on nursing students' academic performance. Richards (1977) conducted a 3-year study of 250 entering and graduating students in a 4-year baccalaureate nursing program, including one class of students who completed a traditional block program and two classes of students who completed a new integrated curriculum. The study was part of a commitment by the faculty to examine the curriculum and its products, the students. Students were assessed in terms of their personality characteristics, intelligence, initial thinking, and empathic ability. Knowledge of nursing was measured using clinical grade-point averages, state board examination scores, and scores on the medical–surgical, psychiatric, public health, pediatric, and obstetric nursing sections of the National League for Nursing (NLN) examination.

Study results related to parent–child nursing indicated that students in the integrated curriculum scored significantly higher on the pediatric portion of the NLN examination than did students in the block curriculum. On the obstetric portion of the NLN examination, mean scores were lowest for students at the end of the second year of the integrated curriculum and highest for students at the end of the first year of the integrated curriculum, with the scores for students graduating from the block program falling in the middle. However, differences were not significant.

On state board examinations, students graduating from the integrated curriculum had lower mean scores in both pediatrics and obstetrics than students completing the block curriculum. The difference was significant only for the pediatric scores. The researchers reported that these results were "nonconclusive" in terms of the knowledge base of students in the block and integrated programs but emphasized that it was clear that students in both programs met standards for licensure. The results of the study also indicated that obstetric and pediatric scores on state board examinations could be predicted best by a combination of NLN scores and the nursing grade-point average (GPA), accounting for 68% of the variance in obstetric scores and 72% of the variance in pediatric scores. Students in the integrated curriculum tended to demonstrate a higher degree of leadership and empathic ability than did students in the block curriculum but had less critical thinking ability. Richards (1977) made a substantive effort to measure a number of outcomes as a nursing program changed its curricular structure from a block model to an integrated model. However, without an analysis of how the processes and emphases of nursing education changed, interpretation of the results is difficult.

Teaching methods, clinical experiences, and the placement of parent–child nursing in undergraduate nursing programs have been the subject of several studies. Fouts and Fogel (1980) examined teaching methods and clinical experiences utilized by baccalaureate nursing programs in teaching obstetrical and gynecological nursing. A brief questionnaire asking for information about lecture presentation, textbooks, clinical experiences, supervision, and program statistics was mailed to all baccalaureate nursing programs ($N = 309$). Two hundred and two questionnaires were returned representing schools with 2-, 3-, and 4-year professional programs.

Results of the study indicated that most obstetrical theory was placed in the junior year, with content hours varying widely. More than half of the programs presented content in a block rather than integrated fashion. A wide variety of textbooks, methods, and clinical experiences were reported. Although approximately half of the 2- and 3-year professional programs indicated a preference not to present content in large groups, over half (58%) of the 4-year schools reported using the large-group format. Clinical experiences in all three types of programs were offered largely in block form and in both inpatient and outpatient facilities. Short-term intensive experiences with both mother and infant and long-term experience with the pregnant family seemed to be essential. Faculty–student ratios varied from 1:8 to 1:10. The trend appeared to be for students in inpatient settings to have direct faculty supervision, whereas supervision was indirect in outpatient settings. In general, little emphasis was placed by schools on gynecologic content or clinical experience. Although the study was exploratory in design and designed only to describe strategies used by baccalaureate nursing programs in teaching obstetric and gynecologic content, the authors suggested the need for future examination of the rationale for these selected strategies.

Sherwen and Raff (1987) surveyed maternal–infant curricula and teaching methods used in NLN-accredited baccalaureate nursing (BSN) programs. A pilot study was conducted of 50 representative BSN programs to determine the placement and content of maternal–infant curricular information. Four models were identified: the childbearing-rearing family model (54% of programs); the block "Big 5" medical model (14% of programs); the integrated model (21% of programs); and the nurse-theoretician model (11% of programs). Twenty-three percent of the programs surveyed supplemented maternal–infant content with independent learning aids. One program offered a senior elective in advanced high-risk maternity nursing. Although the time allotted to maternal–infant nursing varied widely, there seemed to be a progression from normal maternal experience to high-risk experience. Only 11% of the programs incorporated women's health or gynecologic content into maternal and child health courses. Although purely descriptive in nature, the study findings supported the trend for baccalaureate nursing programs to offer maternal–infant content in broader-focused, more integrated models. The authors reported that this study was preliminary to a larger core competency project.

The most comprehensive project exploring parent–child nursing education thus far is the 3-year Maternal Infant Core Competency Project. This project represents a joint effort among the March of Dimes Foundation, The American Association of Colleges of Nursing, the Nurses' Association of the American College of Obstetrics and Gynecology, and the American Nurses' Association. The goal was to develop a core competency framework for the maternal–infant component in baccalaureate nursing education. The project was funded by the Division of Maternal and Child Health, U.S. Public Health Service, Department of Health and Human Services.

Sherwen (1987) reported on Phase I of the project, which was a national survey of maternal–infant nurse educators and practicing nurses from acute-care and community health settings. Two instruments were pilot-tested and used in the study: one instrument for nurse educators, and one for practitioners. Respondents provided information concerning perceptions of what content ideally should be taught and at what level, as well as what actually was being taught and its level. Respondents included 364 faculty from 202 NLN-accredited baccalaureate nursing programs across the country and 126 practicing nurses, half of whom were practicing in community health settings, with the remainder in acute care settings.

Analysis of the data revealed that within both educator and practitioner groups there were statistically significant differences between what were perceived as ideal and real situations. Nursing educators perceived that maternal–infant nursing content and skills should be taught at a higher level than was practiced currently by baccalaureate nursing students. Nursing practitioners perceived that the ideal level at which maternal–infant content and skills should be taught to baccalaureate nursing students was higher than the level at which the content and skills actually were demonstrated by new graduates. When the educators and practitioners were compared with each other, there was considerable agreement on maternal–infant content that should be included in the ideal baccalaureate program, but not on the level at which it should be taught. Educators apparently thought that content should be taught at a higher level than did practicing nurses. Sherwen (1987) concluded that nursing faculty may have unrealistically high expectations of the level at which maternal–infant content should be taught to baccalaureate nursing students and that, in fact, practicing nurses do not expect this high level of performance of new graduates, nor do they actually see it.

Through this first phase of the Maternal–Infant Core Competency Project significant strides have been made in quantifying differences within and between nursing education and nursing practice on perceptions of the level at which critical maternal–infant core competency should be taught. The project also has highlighted the need for further dialogue between maternal–infant nursing educators and practitioners. However, some confusion remains. It would seem appropriate not only to delineate competencies expected of the baccalaureate graduate but also to examine those expected of the master's student with specialty preparation in the maternal–infant area. Such an examination of a "progression" of competencies from the baccalaureate through the master's level would go a long way toward addressing some of the ambiguities that now exist.

Studies of parent–child nursing curricula at the baccalaureate level have not been analytic but rather have been focused largely on simple descriptions of the way in which content and clinical experiences are structured in the relationship between academic preparation and competency in clinical practice. The one possible exception is the Maternal–Infant Core Competency Project (Sherwen, 1987), in which attempts were made to articulate the perceptions of nurse educators and practitioners about what maternal–infant content should be taught and the level at which it should be taught. What can be gleaned with some confidence from these studies is how parent–child nursing content is being taught and, to a lesser degree, what is being taught, but not what should be taught given current parent–child health issues.

Graduate Nursing Curricula

Keppler, DeMoya, Murchland, Pyne, and Terrell (1977) were concerned about acute shortages of professional nurses specializing in maternal–child nursing and surveyed all ($N = 200$) graduate nursing students in a large university program, excluding those students in maternal and child health. The study instrument, developed and piloted by the researchers, was designed to gather information in the areas of personal background, work experience, and prior education and learning experiences, especially in maternal and child care.

The results of the survey revealed no factor of particular importance in the students' basic maternal–child nursing educational background that would lead to its exclusion as an area of specialization at the graduate level. More than half of the students surveyed described their undergraduate maternal–child nursing instructors in negative terms. Nurses who worked outside the maternal–child nursing area appeared to be in their positions by choice, whereas those working in maternal–child units reported that they were in their positions by assignment. Those employed in maternal–child units also reported having had less orientation to the clinical area. This study was limited in scope and design and included only students in one graduate nursing program. Further research is needed about graduate nursing students' reasons for choosing *not* to specialize in maternal–child health, as well as their reasons for choosing that field of study.

McKevitt (1986) was interested in identifying trends in master's-level graduate nursing education programs over the 5 years from 1979 to 1984. The sample for the study included all NLN-accredited master's programs listed in the NLN publication *Masters Education in Nursing: Route to Opportunities in Contemporary Nursing* (NLN, 1979, 1983) for the years 1979–1980 ($N = 81$ programs) and 1983–1984 ($N = 118$ programs). Data were derived from information about the program listed in the NLN publication and from college and university catalogs and brochures. The results of the study indicated that in 1979 there were 95 maternal– or parent–child health majors within 57 programs, whereas in 1984 there were 171 majors within 82 programs. Specialty majors in maternal and child health outnumbered general majors in 1979 and 1984. Within the specialty majors, growth was greatest in the areas of perinatal/neonatal nursing, women's health, children's and adolescents' health, and primary care pediatrics. Although addressing only NLN-accredited programs, the study results suggested an increasing trend toward the division of parent–child nursing content into specialized, narrowly defined areas.

Williamson (1983) conducted a similar review of NLN-accredited master's programs. Based on an examination of the NLN publication *Master's Education in Nursing: Route to Opportunities in Contemporary Nursing 1982–83* (NLN, 1982), Williamson identified more than 130 words or phrases used to describe clinical areas of study. Functional components were not considered. Grouping what appeared to be similar clinical areas of study, the author identified 14 groups, over half of which seem to include areas related to maternal and child health. In spite of the somewhat arbitrary assignment of clinical areas of study to groups, it was clear that both this author and McKevitt (1986) reported similar findings, a plethora of parent–child-related graduate nursing majors. Williamson (1983) suggested that consensus is needed in academic nomenclature in graduate nursing education, emphasizing consistency of purpose and clear communication.

Studies of parent–child nursing curricula at the graduate level have done little more than support the notion that there are a variety of graduate nursing programs that are in some way related to parent–child health. There were no studies in which investigators began to define what was included or should be included in graduate-level preparation in these programs, that is, what constitutes advanced preparation in parent–child nursing. Much research remains to be done.

PREDICTING SUCCESS ON STATE BOARD TEST EXAMINATIONS

Thirteen studies were designed to identify predictors of state board examination performance. In all studies but one, researchers used descriptive designs. Diploma graduates served as subjects for one study (Shelley, Kennamer, & Raile, 1976), associate degree students as subjects for five studies (Backman & Steindler, 1971; Deardorff, Denner, & Miller, 1976; Papcum, 1971; Reed & Feldhusen, 1972; Wolfle & Bryant, 1978), and baccalaureate graduates as subjects for six studies (Bell & Martindell, 1976; Melcolm, Venn, & Bausell, 1981; Muhlenkamp, 1971; Perez, 1977; Stronk, 1972; Yocum & Scherubel, 1985). In one study, the state board examination performance for all three types of nursing graduates was compared (McQuaid & Kane, 1979).

Several predictors were investigated with some regularity across studies: performance on the NLN achievement tests (Bell & Martindell, 1976; Melcolm et al., 1981; Muhlenkamp, 1971; Richards, 1977; Shelley, et al., 1976); overall college grade-point average (GPA) as well as grade-point averages in specific college courses (Perez, 1977; Stronk, 1972; Wolfle & Bryant, 1978; Yocum & Scherubel, 1985); the Scholastic Aptitude Test (SAT) (Backman & Steindler, 1971; Muhlenkamp, 1971; Reed & Feldhusen, 1972; Wolfle & Bryant, 1978); and nursing theory and clinical grades (Muhlenkamp, 1971). Predictors such as high school class rank (Backman & Steindler, 1971) and standardized aptitude tests (Perez, 1977; Wolfle & Bryant, 1978) appeared less frequently.

It is difficult to draw conclusions about the role played by parent–child nursing education on state board examination performance, given the diversity of predictor variables examined and the variety of research methodologies used. In general, predictors of performance in the medical, surgical, and psychiatric components of the state board examination were similar to those predicting pediatric or obstetrical nursing state board performance.

A few exceptions bear note. In a study of 51 baccalaureate graduates, Muhlenkamp (1971) found that the NLN Science Test was the best predictor of state board performance for all of the components except pediatric nursing. For this component, the seventh-semester grade-point average and the NLN Maternal and Child Achievement Test explained the greatest variation in state board scores. Similar findings were reported by Melcolm et al. (1981). These researchers identified predictors of state board performance for graduates of an integrated nursing curriculum. Subjects were 390 baccalaureate graduates of the 1976 and 1977 classes at the University of Maryland School of Nursing. Results on the NLN Maternal and Child Achievement Test along with Part A of the NLN Medical–Surgical Achievement Test demonstrated the highest correlations ($r = .56$) with pediatric nursing state board scores. When other NLN achievement test scores and nursing theory and clinical grades for the junior and senior years were controlled in a series of stepwise multiple regression equations, the Nursing of Children Achievement Test was consistently either the second- or third-best predictor of variation in state board scores for each of the state board components. No explanation was given for this finding.

Wolfle and Bryant (1978) used a causal model to assess relationships among a variety of predictor variables and state board examination performance. They hypothesized that academic ability and college achievement influenced state board test performance directly as well as indirectly through effects on NLN achievement scores. Academic ability was measured by SAT verbal and quantitative scores. College achievement was assessed by overall undergraduate grade-point average. Data for testing this model came from all graduates of an associate degree nursing program in southwest Virginia from 1970 and 1976. The investigators found that one fifth of the relationship between medical, surgical, and obstetric nursing NLN test scores and state board examination scores was attributed to the student's academic ability and college achievement. In contrast, a full two fifths of the relationship between scores on NLN achievement tests and state board examinations for pediatrics and psychiatric nursing were traceable to academic ability and college achievement. Students with high academic abilities performed well on both examinations, leading the researchers to conclude that success in pediatric and psychiatric nursing examinations was more a function of general ability than mastery of subject matter. It was unclear to what extent the content of these examinations influenced the findings. If the content tested in pediatric and psychiatric nursing examinations drew heavily on logical thinking and decision making, then it is not surprising that measures of aptitude and achievement in college courses would correlate with successful performance.

PREDICTING SUCCESS IN GRADUATE NURSING PROGRAMS

Measures of academic achievement (grade-point average) and aptitude (Graduate Record Examination) have served as the primary predictors of success in graduate-level nursing programs. Studies have been focused on grade-point averages in nursing and nonnursing courses as outcomes (Sime, 1978; Thomas, 1977; Tripp & Duffey, 1981). Only a few studies were addressed to the criteria that predict success for various clinical specialties.

Data from a sample of 198 master's-degree graduates of medical–surgical nursing, nursing of children, psychiatric nursing, and nursing administration programs at the University of Iowa (1972–1975) were analyzed to examine the effectiveness of undergraduate grade-point average (GPA) and Graduate Record Examination (GRE) verbal and quantitative scores in predicting graduate level GPA. The undergraduate GPA was the strongest predictor of graduate GPA for students in the nursing of children clinical specialty. Overall, predictors operated differently for the four nursing specialties, indicating that differential weights should be applied in assessing the academic success of graduate nursing students (Thomas, 1977).

Munro (1985) used a combination of record and interview data in an investigation of criteria that predict success in graduate clinical specialty programs. Information was gathered from the records of 435 master's-degree nurses at Yale University from 1974 through 1981. Grade-point averages for nursing theory courses, clinical courses, and total courses were regressed on six predictors: GRE verbal scores, GRE quantitative scores, undergraduate GPA, the quality of the student's application essay, ratings of the student at the time of interview for graduate school, and ratings provided by references. For the pediatric clinical specialty program, GRE verbal scores produced the highest correlations with the overall GPA ($r = .42$), followed by GRE quantitative scores ($r = .33$) and ratings by references ($r = .33$). In total, the six predictors accounted for only 8 to 10% of the variation in graduate grade-point averages for any of the clinical specialty programs. None of the predictors was associated significantly with the grade-point average in clinical coursework. These findings support the work of Sime (1978), Stein and Green (1970), and Ainslie et al. (1976), who suggested that the Graduate Record Examination had little significant predictive value for performance in nursing courses.

In these studies, the Graduate Record Examination correlated more sharply with nonnursing than with nursing course performance. Despite small samples, this finding across studies raises questions about the use of the GRE as a predictor of success in graduate programs in nursing. It may be that the complexity of reasoning required in graduate nursing courses is not assessed easily by tests of verbal and quantitative abilities. Achievement tests in clinical areas may serve as stronger predictors of success in graduate nursing programs (Stein & Green, 1970).

SUMMARY AND FUTURE RESEARCH DIRECTIONS

Research was presented under two major categories: studies related to undergraduate and graduate nursing curricula, and studies designed to predict success on state board examinations or in graduate clinical specialty programs. A critical review of the published research yielded little information about the efficacy of parent–child nursing education. Indeed, more questions were raised than were answered as a result of this review.

Studies of undergraduate curricula gave evidence that shifts occurred in parent–child nursing content as baccalaureate programs moved from a medical model to an integrated curriculum during the mid-1970s. Unfortunately, few researchers have investigated the impact of the integrated curriculum on academic performance in parent–child nursing courses or on clinical practice behavior. Only four descriptive studies were identified in which content issues were addressed. Of these, the Maternal–Infant Core Competency Project (Sherwen, 1987) seemed to hold the greatest promise for clarifying content and competency in parent–child nursing.

Despite recent growth in the numbers of parent–child graduate nursing programs, there is a dearth of research on the impact of these programs on advanced clinical nursing practice. The published literature continues to focus attention on academic achievement in graduate school while remaining silent on such programmatic outcomes of graduate nursing education as changes in parent–child nursing practice or patient care. Such investigations are challenging, requiring longitudinal data and measurable behavioral outcomes. At a minimum, it would be useful to have descriptive studies of the kinds of positions master's-prepared parent–child nurses hold as well as evaluation of how well they perceive their graduate education provided preparation for their jobs.

In the 1970s, findings in studies of state board examination performance indicated few differences between predictors of success in the pediatric and obstetric components of the examination and those for medical, surgical, and psychiatric nursing components. NLN Achievement Test scores and overall grade-point averages have a documented association with state board examination (SBE) performance, whereas pediatric or obstetric nursing course grades consistently have been poor predictors of state board success. Findings in more recent studies of graduates from programs with integrated nursing curricula further confirmed the limitations in use of clinical and nursing theory course grades as predictors of SBE scores. The recent implementation of a national state board examination with an overall score negates future use of SBE performance as an outcome for parent–child nursing education.

In part, research in parent–child nursing education at both undergraduate and graduate levels has been hampered by definitional ambiguities. What was simply obstetric or pediatric nursing 15 years ago has become maternal and child nursing, parent and child nursing, family nursing, perinatal health, or women's health. The enormity of the field coupled with an absence of standard nomenclature for defining its parameters places severe limitations on the development of core content and core clinical competencies.

The regionalization of perinatal services in the late 1970s may have contributed to the increasing specialization in parent–child nursing, especially at the graduate level. With high-risk mothers and infants concentrated in tertiary-care hospitals, the need for nurses with highly specialized clinical skills grew at a time when parent–child nursing programs were moving to integrated curricula. Thus, the development of specialties in parent–child nursing education may have been a response to both changes in nursing curricula and broad technological changes in the delivery of health care to mothers and children.

Before studies can be designed to address the impact of parent–child educational programs on nursing practice, it is important to establish standard nomenclature for defining the field. As a second step, research is needed to identify and delineate core content areas and clinical competencies at both undergraduate and graduate levels. Only after parameters are defined and content areas delineated can investigators begin to document empirically the impact of education on parent–child nursing practice.

REFERENCES

Ainslie, B., Andersen, L., Colby, B. K., Hoffman, M. A., Meserve, K. P., O'Connor, C., & Ouimet, K. (1976). Predictive value of selected admission criteria for graduate nursing education. *Nursing Research, 25,* 296–299.

Backman, M., & Steindler, F. (1971). Prediction of achievement in a collegiate nursing program and performance on state board examinations. *Nursing Outlook, 19,* 487.

Bell, J., & Martindell, C. (1976). Cross-validation study for predictors of scores on state board examinations. *Nursing Research, 25,* 54–57.

Deardorff, M., Denner, P., & Miller, C. A. (1976). Selected National League for Nursing achievement test scores as predictors of state board examination scores. *Nursing Research, 25,* 35–38.

Fouts, J., & Fogel, C. (1980). A survey of obstetrical teaching strategies in baccalaureate schools of nursing. *Journal of Nursing Education, 19*(7), 18–26.

Keppler, A., DeMoya, D., Murchland, A., Pyne, H., & Terrell, E. (1977). Where are the maternal–child nursing graduate students? *Journal of Obstetric, Gynecologic and Neonatal Nursing, 6*(6), 27–30.

McKevitt, R. K. (1986). Trends in master's education in nursing. *Journal of Professional Nursing, 2,* 225–233.

McQuaid, E., & Kane, M. (1979). How do graduates of different types of programs perform on state boards? *American Journal of Nursing, 79,* 305–308.

Melcolm, N., Venn, R., & Bausell, R. B. (1981). The prediction of state board test pool examination scores within an integrated curriculum. *Journal of Nursing Education, 20*(5), 24–28.

Muhlenkamp, A. (1971). Prediction of state board scores in a baccalaureate program. *Nursing Outlook, 19,* 57.

Munro, B. (1985). Predicting success in graduate clinical specialty programs. *Nursing Research, 34,* 54–57.

National League for Nursing, Division of Baccalaureate and Higher Degree Programs. (1979). *Master's Education in Nursing: Route to Opportunities in*

Contemporary Nursing 1979–1980 (Pub. No. 15-1312). New York: Author.

National League for Nursing, Division of Baccalaureate and Higher Degree Programs. (1982). *Master's Education in Nursing: Route to Opportunities in Contemporary Nursing 1982–1983* (Pub. No. 15-1312). New York: Author.

National League for Nursing, Division of Baccalaureate and Higher Degree Programs. (1983). *Master's Education in Nursing: Route to Opportunities in Contemporary Nursing 1983–84* (Pub. No. 15-1312). New York: Author.

Papcum, I. D. (1971). Results of achievement tests and state board tests in an associate degree program. *Nursing Outlook, 19,* 341.

Perez, T. (1977). Investigation of academic moderator variables to predict success on state board of nursing examinations in a baccalaureate nursing program. *Journal of Nursing Education, 16*(8), 16–23.

Reed, C., & Feldhusen, J. (1972). State board examination score prediction for associate degree nursing program graduates. *Nursing Research, 21,* 149–153.

Richards, M. A. (1977). One integrated curriculum: An empirical evaluation. *Nursing Research, 26,* 90–95.

Shelley, B., Kennamer, D., & Raile, M. (1976). Correlations of NLN achievement test scores with state board test pool examination scores. *Nursing Outlook, 24,* 52–55.

Sherwen, L. N. (1987). The maternal–infant core competency project: Report of phase I. *Journal of Professional Nursing, 3,* 230–241.

Sherwen, L. N., & Raff, B. (1987). Maternal–infant core competencies in the BSN curricula. *American Journal of Nursing, 3,* 845–846.

Sime, A. (1978). Prediction of success in a master's program in nursing. *Psychological Reports, 42,* 779–783.

Stein, K., & Green, E. (1970). The graduate record examination as a predictive potential in the nursing major. *Nursing Research, 19,* 42–47.

Stronk, D. (1972). Predicting student performance from college admission criteria. *Nursing Outlook, 27,* 604–607.

Thomas, B. (1977). Differential utility of predictors in graduate nursing education. *Nursing Research, 26,* 100–102.

Tripp, A., & Duffey, M. (1981). Discriminant analysis to predict graduates—nongraduates in a master's degree program in nursing. *Research in Nursing and Health, 4,* 345–353.

Williamson, J. A. (1983). Master's education: A need for nomenclature. *Image, 15,* 99–101.

Wolfle, L., & Bryant, L. (1978). A causal model of nursing education and state board examination scores. *Nursing Research, 27,* 311–315.

Yocum, C., & Scherubel, J. (1985). Selected preadmission and academic correlates of success on state board examinations. *Journal of Nursing Education, 24,* 244–249.

PART IV

Research on the Profession of Nursing

Chapter 9

Moral Reasoning and Ethical Practice

SHAKÉ KETEFIAN
UNIVERSITY OF MICHIGAN

CONTENTS

Recent nursing literature reflects concern over the ethical dimensions of scientific and technological developments. Nurse investigators in greater numbers than ever are engaged in empirical studies of ethical practice. The goal of this integrative review is to infer generalizations

The author wishes to acknowledge the assistance of Ingrid Ormond, a doctoral student at the University of Michigan School of Nursing, who served as research assistant during the preparation of this review. Readers may obtain from the author a summary table, "Instruments to Measure Moral Reasoning and Ethical Practice."

about the substantive issues in research on nurses' moral reasoning and ethical practice. The specific purposes are to: (a) present, analyze, and synthesize research related to moral reasoning and ethical practice; (b) contribute to creating a comprehensible literature in nursing ethics; and (c) suggest directions for future research.

Only one previous review of nursing ethics research was located (Gortner, 1985). Gortner provided a broad examination of ethical inquiry in nursing, covering the period 1968 through 1983. Some discussion of literature was presented in which the nurse (behavior, education, decision making) was the unit of analysis, and measurement of ethics-relevant constructs was identified as an issue of concern.

DEFINITION OF CONSTRUCTS

The constructs of *moral reasoning* and *ethical practice* have not been defined consistently and distinguished from one another in the nursing literature. Moral reasoning refers to the cognitive and developmental process of reasoning about moral choice. The terms *moral judgment* or *moral development* are used commonly in the literature as synonyms for moral reasoning. Ethical practice refers to the decisions made and actions taken in ethical dilemma situations. *Moral behavior, ethical behavior,* and *ethical decision making* commonly are used as synonyms.

Nomenclature is important as one tries to attain clarity of meaning and understanding of the conceptual underpinnings of the studies reviewed. It is important that a construct be operationalized to match the conceptual definition as closely as possible. The matter of nomenclature presents special difficulties with respect to the domains under consideration in the present chapter, as will become evident.

SCOPE OF THE LITERATURE REVIEWED

The population for study was the research literature on moral reasoning and ethical practice published from 1983 through early 1987. This review began in 1983 because Gortner's (1985) previous review on ethical inquiry included the published literature through early 1983. Because of a paucity of published research, dissertations were included.

Published nursing research was identified using a MEDLINE computer search and manual searches of the *Cumulative Index to Nursing and Allied Health Literature;* the journals *Nursing Research, Research in Nursing and Health, Western Journal of Nursing Research,* and *Advances in Nursing Science;* the National League for Nursing publication *Ethics in Nursing: An Annotated Bibliography* (Pence, 1986); and the *Subject Guide to Books in Print 1985–1986* (1985). Also, works were identified by tracking citations in the identified studies. Nursing doctoral dissertations were identified by a University Microfilms International (UMI) Data Direct computer search and by manual review of *Dissertation Abstracts International,* UMI's *Nursing: A Catalog of Selected Doctoral Dissertation Research 1982–1985,* and UMI's 1986 quarterly issues of *Nursing Dissertation Quarterly Update.* Because the number of potential studies was small, all quantitative and qualitative studies conducted by nurse investigators and related to the focus of the review were included.

The studies reviewed might be characterized as being in the domain of descriptive ethics. The descriptive domain is focused on empirical questions of what is, or what people do, think, or believe. A basic assumption underlying descriptive ethics research is that moral judgments frequently draw upon factual beliefs or claims about the world, or presuppose views about the facts of a situation. Research into descriptive ethics thus can serve a highly useful purpose in moral debate by providing factual information and accurate scientific description of a situation.

Excluded from this review were philosophical investigations, unpublished materials, and works in progress. Literature in the domain of normative ethics was not included either. Normative ethics is prescriptive and pertains to questions of what is right or good, how one should behave, and what ought to be the case. Such value questions defy empirical study and are treated through philosophical analysis.

ANALYSIS AND INTERPRETATION

Given the diversity of study foci, methods, and measures, the data analysis procedures of listing and voting were utilized (Cooper, 1982;

Ganong, 1987; Jackson, 1980). Listing entailed specifying those factors that were related across studies to moral reasoning or ethical practice. Voting entailed enumerating the number of studies with positive, negative, and nonsignificant findings regarding a particular research hypothesis. The voting process was focused on results for the main hypotheses of the studies. Findings were reviewed selectively in a few cases in which auxiliary data analyses contributed to understanding of the relationship of the major identified factors to the criterion variables.

Interpretation and discussion are based on the listing and voting method. Compelling positive or negative results are highlighted in the section "Conclusions and Future Directions", and relevant interpretation is provided. Some overall trends are identified regarding knowledge yield and recommendations for future research directions. Although this process was carried out utilizing the objective rules established, it must be acknowledged that the biases of the author may have played a role.

MORAL REASONING

The majority of investigators have used Kohlberg's (1978) theory of moral development to define moral reasoning conceptually. Moral reasoning is defined by Kohlberg as a cognitive and developmental process characterized by the sequential transformation of the way in which social arrangements are interpreted. Also, Kohlberg has defined three successive levels of moral reasoning, with each level consisting of two stages. These levels are: (a) preconventional (stages 1 and 2), in which externally established rules determine right or wrong action; (b) conventional (stages 3 and 4), in which expectations of family and group are maintained, and loyalty and conformity to the existing social order are considered important; and (c) postconventional or principled (stages 5 and 6), in which the individual autonomously examines and defines moral values and principles apart from the group norms of the culture, with decisions of conscience dictating the right action. Each stage is an organized system of thought within which individuals consistently function in their moral judgments. The stages constitute an invariant sequence from simple thought to complex moral reasoning, and the thought processes involved in higher levels of moral development incorporate intellectual tools derived from earlier levels (Rest, 1974a). Each stage is characterized by distinctive ways in which dilemmas and crucial issues are evaluated (Rest, 1976). Kohlberg's (1971, 1978) formulation on moral development has extended the works of Dewey (1964) and Piaget (1965).

In recent years Kohlberg's (1978) conceptualization of moral reasoning has been challenged on the grounds that it reflects a male-oriented perspective of morality. According to Gilligan (1982), women tend to see morality in the context of particular relationships, which she called the "ethic of care." Gilligan argued further that a conception of morality as justice—viewed in terms of obligations and rights, fairness, and impartiality—depicts a male view and obscures female reality. Kohlberg, Levine, and Hewer (1984) conceded that conceiving of morality in terms of justice has led to the design of Kohlberg's Moral Judgment Interview, which is focused on conflicting rights and distribution of scarce resources, and that these foci do not include concern for others or areas other than justice that are part of the moral domain.

Measurement

Two main measures, the Defining Issues Test (Rest, 1974b) and the Nursing Dilemma Test (Crisham, 1981), were utilized by the investigators included in this review. Nine investigators used the Defining Issues Test, one used the Nursing Dilemma Test, three used both tests, and one used an investigator-modified version of the Defining Issues Test. A third measure, the Moral Judgment Interview (Colby, Kohlberg, Gibbs, Candee, Speicher-Dubin, & Hewer, 1983), was used once.

Moral Judgment Interview. The Moral Judgment Interview (MJI) requires subjects to generate verbalizations in response to open-ended questions, and is focused on situations of conflicting rights and distribution of scarce resources (Colby, Kohlberg, Gibbs, & Lieberman, 1983; Kohlberg et al., 1984). The Interview scoring procedure results in assigning a subject to a stage of moral reasoning. Because a respondent is not credited with an idea unless it is articulated clearly, the level of moral development can be underestimated. Over the years, the MJI has been refined and its validity and reliability enhanced. Intensive training is required to administer, code, and score the Interview reliably. The Moral Judgment Interview has had a profound effect on other measures of moral reasoning.

Defining Issues Test. The Defining Issues Test (DIT) is a multiple choice, objective, self-administered tool based on Kohlberg's theory of moral development (Rest, 1974b, 1976, 1979). The respondent is required to rank stage-relevant statements. The test yields two indices: the P score and the D score. Both indices are continuous measures. The P score represents principled thinking, whereas the D score represents the relative preference for principled thinking over conventional and pre-conventional reasoning. The DIT also can be scored in a manner that enables stage-typing subjects. This procedure is utilized less frequently.

Correlations as high as .68 have been reported between the Defining Issues Test and the Moral Judgment Interview (Rest, 1975a, 1975b). However, more recent investigators have reported low correlations (.24, .35) between the DIT and MJI (Bode & Page, 1978; Davidson & Robbins, 1978; Kay, 1982).

Nursing Dilemma Test. The Nursing Dilemma Test is a measure of moral reasoning in nursing situations and is based on the Defining Issues Test (Crisham, 1981). The Nursing Dilemma Test measures two additional dimensions: nurses' degree of familiarity with similar dilemmas and the relative importance given to practical considerations in making decisions on moral issues. Crisham has reported a positive correlation between the Defining Issues Test and the Nursing Dilemma Test, but the correlation magnitude is not provided. The coefficient alpha for the principled nursing considerations (NP) score is estimated as .57 (Crisham, 1981).

Study Characteristics

Investigators have used various research designs and samples to examine moral reasoning. Three studies were experimental or quasi-experimental (S. K. Bell, 1984; Frisch, 1986; Kellmer, 1984); seven were descriptive-correlational (Aronovitz, 1984; Beardslee, 1983; de Jong, 1985; Felton, 1984; Fleeger, 1986; Gaul, 1987b; Mustapha, 1985); four were descriptive-exploratory (Forman, 1986; Holzman, 1984; Mayberry, 1983; Winland-Brown, 1983); and one was descriptive-qualitative (Omery, 1986). A majority of investigators used nursing students, most often baccalaureate students, as samples; a minority used practicing nurses.

Researchers have addressed several predictor variables in a number of studies, respectively: academic level, academic major, or type of program ($n = 8$); ethics course or curriculum content related to ethics ($n = 4$); cognitive development, critical thinking, or intelligence ($n = 4$); religion ($n = 4$); age ($n = 4$); grade-point average and Scholastic

Aptitude Test scores ($n = 3$); prior clinical or work experience ($n = 3$); area of practice ($n = 3$); socioeconomic status ($n = 3$); and gender ($n = 2$). A number of other variables were used only once. The studies suffered from a number of methodological shortcomings. A majority of investigators used convenience samples; when different groups were employed for comparison purposes, no effort was made to obtain adequate-sized groups for comparisons. Many failed to control for preexisting group differences or for relevant intervening variables. A number of investigators analyzed results at such a level of specificity that broad trends were difficult to discern. Examples of such analysis included testing hypotheses for each of the six dilemma situations in the Nursing Dilemma Test or the Defining Issues Test, or reporting results for each moral development level or stage. Despite these shortcomings, the collective findings have been examined for important trends.

Findings

Education.   Kohlberg (1978) has posited that moral development is influenced by education. Education, when structured to create cognitive conflict and disequilibrium by showing inadequacies in a person's mode of thinking, is believed to stimulate individuals to seek higher and more adequate ways to reason about moral choice (Rest, Turiel, & Kohlberg, 1969). However, no relationship between nursing students' educational level and moral reasoning was found by three investigators (Aronovitz, 1984; Fleeger, 1986; Mustapha, 1985); Felton reported a positive relationship of educational level with the Defining Issues Test D score, but not with the P score (Felton, 1984; Felton & Parsons, 1987). Holzman (1984) reported a negative relationship and nursing undergraduate students had lower moral reasoning scores than other undergraduate students (Holzman, 1984; Mustapha, 1985). The relationship between nurses' educational level and moral reasoning was reported, respectively, as positive, negative, and nonsignificant (Gaul, 1987b; Mayberry, 1983, 1986; Winland-Brown, 1983).

Results were inconclusive for the relationship between ethics instruction and moral reasoning. One investigator reported higher moral reasoning following an ethics course (S. K. Bell, 1984); another reported a higher Defining Issues Test stage score but no differences on Defining Issues Test P score or Nursing Dilemma Test scores between instructed and control groups (Frisch, 1986); and a third investigator reported no difference between instructed and control groups (Kellmer, 1984). The level of ethics content in baccalaureate nursing curriculums was unrelated to moral reasoning (Beardslee, 1983).

Cognitive Variables. Kohlberg (1971) proposed that intellectual development influenced the level of moral development. People capable of processing information at the level of formal operations were expected to be more advanced in their moral development than those at the level of concrete thought. Investigators reported that several cognitive variables were related positively to moral reasoning. The cognitive variables included critical thinking (Fleeger, 1986), intelligence (de Jong, 1985; Mustapha, 1985), college grade-point average (Fleeger, 1986; Mustapha, 1985), and scores on the Scholastic Aptitude Test (SAT) (Fleeger, 1986; Mustapha, 1985). No relationships with moral reasoning were found for cognitive development (Frisch, 1986) or high school grade-point average (Fleeger, 1986).

Different results were reported for the various moral reasoning measures. Mustapha (1985) reported that variance in the Defining Issues Test P score (12%), but not the D score, was explained by the combination of intelligence and grade-point average; also, variance in the P score (10%), but not the D score, was explained by the SAT. College grade-point average was correlated positively with the D but not the P score (Fleeger, 1986); nursing grade-point average, cumulative grade-point average, and age together explained 30% of the variance in the Nursing Dilemma Test score (principled nursing considerations), whereas the Defining Issues Test score was not significantly related to those variables (Kellmer, 1984).

Environment. Social climate has been posited by Kohlberg (1971) to affect moral development. Environments that provide opportunities for group participation, shared decision making, and assumption of responsibility for consequences of action are viewed to stimulate the development of higher levels of moral judgment. No social climate variables were examined other than area of practice variables. Staff nurses had higher Defining Issues Test P scores than head nurses, but not D scores (Mayberry, 1983, 1986). Intensive care unit nurses scored higher on two out of six Nursing Dilemma Test dilemmas than medical-surgical nurses (Winland-Brown, 1983); psychiatric and medical nurses did not differ on moral reasoning (Forman, 1986).

Personal Characteristics. Personal characteristics generally were unrelated to moral reasoning. Aronovitz (1984) noted no difference in moral reasoning scores for gender, whereas Mustapha (1985) found that female students scored higher than male students on the Defining Issues Test P score, but not the D score. Age was reported to be related positively to moral reasoning by Kellmer (1984), but not by others (Gaul, 1987b; Mayberry, 1983, 1986; Mustapha, 1985). Socioeconomic status (Aronovitz, 1984; Fleeger, 1986; Mustapha, 1985) and religion (Aronovitz, 1984; Fleeger, 1986; Kellmer, 1984; Mustapha, 1985; Winland-Brown, 1983) were unrelated to moral reasoning. Work experience was noted to be related positively to moral reasoning by Winland-Brown (1983), but not by Kellmer (1984) or Mayberry (1983).

Description of Moral Reasoning.   Moral reasoning was discovered in a qualitative study of intensive care unit nurses (Omery, 1986) to consist of three components: mode of reasoning, principles, and mitigating factors. Two modes of reasoning were identified: sovereign reasoning, in which judgments were based on self-chosen and valued principles regardless of the identified group norm, and accommodating reasoning, in which reasoning was reconciled to conform to the perceived group norm. Omery identified 15 principles used by nurses to justify their decisions and direct their actions and 12 contextual factors that mitigated which principles were applied in a given situation. The mode of reasoning fashioned the rationale and manner by which the principles and mediating factors were implemented.

ETHICAL PRACTICE

The construct of ethical practice has not been conceptualized adequately within the context of professional nursing practice. Nurse investigators have used various nomenclatures and conceptual definitions of ethical practice. An underlying concern appears to have been the nurse's professional responsibility to deal effectively with situations of ethical conflict and ambiguity that arise in nursing practice. In the general literature, moral behavior has been characterized in terms of delinquency, honesty, altruistic behaviors, resistance to conformity, concern for others, responsible behavior, promise keeping, altruistic commitment, and helping a stranger in need (Blasi, 1980; Brown, 1974; Epstein, 1978; Jacobs, 1977; Staub, 1974).

Measurement

The construct of ethical practice was not defined consistently in operational terms. Six investigators used the Judgments About Nursing

Decisions (Ketefian, 1981, 1985) to measure the dependent variable. Most other investigators developed a test of their own for purposes of the study; a few modified existing instruments to suit their study purposes.

Investigator-Constructed Measures. All except one investigator-constructed measure involves written simulations. The typical format is to present a story that depicts a realistic nursing dilemma, followed by a series of questions, depending on the particular study focus. Examples include: how nurses perceive their participation in ethical decision making (Holly, 1986); listing interventions that might represent a specific ethical principle or philosophical orientation (Finch, 1986; Garritson, 1986); listing interventions representing the tenets of the American Nurses' Association (ANA) Code for Nurses (Cox, 1986; Ketefian, 1985); identifying whether a situation poses an ethical dilemma, what to do, and what might have brought it about (Keller, 1985); and identifying the extent to which nurses advocate for clients, physicians, or employers (Pinch, 1985).

One test involved observation of behavior and was developed by Turner (1984), who adapted procedures used by McNamee (1978). The focus was to observe and measure the extent to which a subject offered assistance to an accomplice manifesting emotional problems from use of an illegal drug. A subsequent interview then delved into the reasons for the nurse's exhibited behavior.

Scant attention was given to the validity and reliability of the investigator-constructed measures. Each instrument was used only by the investigator who designed it.

Judgments About Nursing Decisions. The Judgments About Nursing Decisions instrument measures two dimensions of moral behavior: professionally ideal moral behavior (column A) and realistically likely moral behavior (column B), using the Code for Nurses (ANA, 1976, 1985) as the standard for nursing practice (Ketefian, 1981, 1982, 1984). It is a self-administered, objective measure with six stories depicting nurses in ethical dilemmas. Each story is followed by a list of six or seven nursing actions. Respondents indicate whether the nurse experiencing the dilemma in the story should engage in that action (column A) and whether the nurse experiencing the dilemma is likely to engage in the nursing action (column B).

Content validity of the Judgments About Nursing Decisions was established. Cronbach's coefficient alpha for internal consistency of column B for different registered nurse samples ranged from .66 to .73 (Ketefian, 1984). Although the B scale is considered reliable, no direct inference can be made to the respondent's own actions because it measures respondent's beliefs of what the nurse in the situation would do. Reliability for column A is low, and therefore this scale is not recommended for hypothesis testing.

Study Characteristics

The designs used to study ethical practice included: descriptive correlational (Copstead, 1983; Cox, 1986; de Jong, 1985; Felton, 1984; Finch, 1986; Garritson, 1986; Gaul, 1987b; Holly, 1986; Ketefian, 1985; Nokes, 1985; Turner, 1984); descriptive exploratory (Dison, 1986; Keller, 1985; Lawrence & Crisham, 1984; Ott, 1986; Pinch, 1985); experimental or quasi-experimental (Gaul, 1987a; Husted, 1983); and qualitative (Akerlund & Norberg, 1985; C. M. W. Bell, 1983; Swider, McElmurry, & Yarling, 1985; Zablow, 1985). Subjects were practicing nurses from a variety of work settings (15 studies), nursing students (4 studies), and a combination of students and nurses (3 studies).

The number of studies follows in which researchers addressed each of several predictor variables respectively: education level or type ($n = 9$); organizational or social climate, and variables related to the work environment ($n = 7$); moral reasoning ($n = 6$); previous ethics instruction ($n = 4$); and instruction in ethics or ethical decision making ($n = 2$). A number of other variables were used only once.

Methodological weaknesses of these studies were similar to those previously discussed in the review of studies on moral reasoning. The weaknesses included the predominant use of convenience samples and failure to control for relevant intervening variables. The dependent variables were conceptualized poorly as indices of ethical practice, and many of the measures for the dependent variables lacked validity and reliability.

Findings

Given the diverse range of predictors used and the dissimilarities in the definitions and measures used for the ethical practice variables in these studies, generalizations as to what the results mean collectively are difficult to formulate. However, some tentative statements may be possible in the case of groups of studies that had a common focus; these generalizations are addressed below in terms of selected predictors.

Education.   Prevalent in the nursing literature has been the belief that education promotes ethical practice. However, nurses' educational level was unrelated to ethical practice (Cox, 1986; Gaul, 1987b; Holly, 1986; Keller, 1985; Nokes, 1985; Swider, McElmurry, & Yarling, 1985). Nursing students' academic level was related positively to patient-advocate model selection and risk-taking attitude and negatively related to anxiety produced by the dilemma (Pinch, 1985), but was not related to dilemma resolution ability (Felton, 1984). Nursing students were significantly different from hospital nurses on two out of six Nursing Dilemma Test situations (Lawrence & Crisham, 1984).

Two investigators found no difference on ethical practice between nursing students who had received ethics instruction and a control group (Gaul, 1987a; Husted, 1983). However, the posttest Judgments About Nursing Decisions column A and B scores were correlated positively ($r = .87$) in the ethics group, but not in the control group (Gaul, 1987). Previous ethics education was unrelated to nurses' ethical practice (Copstead, 1983; Holly, 1986; Keller, 1985), except for the finding that students with prior ethics education reported 6 out of 25 dilemma issues more frequently and rated 1 out of 25 issues as more important than students with no prior ethics education (Dison, 1986).

Moral Reasoning.   Persons at higher levels of moral reasoning have been assumed to be more likely to act morally than those at lower levels (Munhall, 1980; Murphy, 1977). However, five investigators reported no relationship between moral reasoning and nurses' ethical practice (Cox, 1986; de Jong, 1985; Felton, 1984; Felton & Parsons, 1987; Gaul, 1987b; Nokes, 1985), even when intelligence (de Jong, 1985) and reading comprehension (Nokes, 1985) were controlled; only one investigator found a positive relationship (Turner, 1984). Turner (1984) reported that the moral judgment stage was associated positively with the consistency between nurses' beliefs of the action that they should have taken in a laboratory situation and the action that they actually had taken. In auxiliary analysis, Nokes (1985) noted a positive correlation ($r = .34$) between moral reasoning and moral behavior when reading comprehension was controlled for white nurses but not for black nurses. Sixty-seven percent of the black nurses were educated outside the United States.

Organizational Variables.   Prevalent in the literature has been the speculation that what is considered ideal ethical practice might not be instituted in the realities of the practice setting (Curtin, 1978; Jameton, 1977). Study results provided some support for a relationship between work environment factors and ethical practice. Nurses' perceptions of their work environment were reported to be related to ethical practice by Akerlund and Norberg (1985) and Garritson (1986), but not by Finch (1986) or Keller (1985). Finch noted that demographic variables—age, nursing experience, religion, clinical area, and others—had no effect on this relationship. Perceived powerlessness was related negatively to moral behavior (Cox, 1986), whereas perceived work autonomy was related positively to moral behavior, but only when intelligence was controlled (de Jong, 1985). Social support in the work environment explained 25% of the variance in perceived participation in ethical decision making (Holly, 1986) but was unrelated to moral behavior in a sample of predominantly foreign-born black nurses (Nokes, 1985).

Description of Ethical Practice. Nurses were found to have difficulty defining or describing ethical dilemmas and in choosing an appropriate course of action (Holly, 1986; Keller, 1985; Zablow, 1985). Nurses used the ethical principles of nonmaleficence and beneficence most frequently (Akerlund & Norberg, 1985; Garritson, 1986). The patterns for making professional decisions differed from those for personal decisions (C. M. W. Bell, 1983). The majority of nurses exhibited a bureaucratic rather than a patient or physician orientation in ethical decision making (Holly, 1986; Swider et al., 1985). Professional categorical (actual) role conception was correlated positively ($r = .30$) with moral behavior, professional normative (ideal) role conception was correlated negatively ($r = -.13$), and bureaucratic role conceptions were unrelated (Ketefian, 1985). The combination of professional and bureaucratic categorical role conceptions explained 11.5% of the variance in moral behavior, whereas the combination of professional and bureaucratic normative role conceptions only explained 3% of the variance.

A discrepancy between ideal and realistic moral behavior was noted by several investigators (C. M. W. Bell, 1983; Copstead, 1983; Gaul, 1987a) using the Judgments About Nursing Decisions instrument: realistic moral behavior was less ANA Code congruent than ideal behavior. In the do not resuscitate decision, Ott (1986) reported that nurses' choice of agent most supportive of patient autonomy was congruent with the investigator's model specification of the agent best able to support patient autonomy. However, a majority of nurses reported that on their units the do not resuscitate decision most likely would be made by a physician rather than the agent they considered to be the most appropriate. C. M. W. Bell (1983) noted that the context of the situation and the consequences associated with the action options influenced nurses' expectations of realistic moral behavior. Ethical situation type was noted by three investigators to influence ethical practice (Husted, 1983; Lawrence & Crisham, 1984; Pinch, 1985); one investigator reported no relationship (Frisch, 1986).

CONCLUSIONS AND FUTURE DIRECTIONS

A number of conclusions are suggested from this integrative review. These are described below.

The relationship between education and moral reasoning remains ambiguous. However, critical thinking, intelligence, grade-point average, and Scholastic Aptitude Test scores are related positively to moral reasoning. It is possible that research design limitations may have obscured the relationship between education and moral reasoning.

One such limitation is the failure of many of the researchers to control for the cognitive variables, such as critical thinking, intelligence, and grade-point average, that relate to moral reasoning. This matter is not simply one of design weakness; possibly nurse investigators fail to appreciate fully the underlying assumptions of the cognitive-developmental theory of moral development. According to this theory, cognitive development is posited as a necessary, though not a sufficient, condition for moral development. Higher-stage thinking typically does not occur developmentally until individuals are well into their twenties. Most investigators have utilized college students who were in their late teens or early twenties; although this choice controls for age, it may have prompted misleading conclusions. The choice of sample and failure to control for cognitive development may have confounded the results in many cases.

An additional limitation relates to measurement issues. Most investigators employed the Defining Issues Test P or D scores. As discussed earlier, the D score is not a recommended measure. Many investigators used the P score to draw conclusions about the stage level of their samples, declaring the majority to be at the conventional level. These conclusions betray a fundamental misunderstanding about the measure. The P index depicts only the postconventional morality level (stages 5 and 6) and yields a continuous score rather than stage-typing subjects. Only two authors (Frisch, 1986; Mayberry, 1983) scored the Defining Issues Test to stage-type subjects. Another feature about the test use relates to a number of built-in reliability and subject consistency checks during scoring. Employing these checks typically results in loss of up to 25 to 30% of the sample; very few authors addressed this feature, and it is not known how many used these rigorous criteria.

Synthesis of findings regarding the effect of some type of teaching program as the intervention on moral reasoning is difficult. The studies were performed using such variation in length, duration, and nature of intervention as to make comparisons across them moot.

The relationship between moral reasoning and moral behavior remained unclear. As presented earlier, five out of six investigators found no relationship between moral reasoning and moral behavior. These findings differed from Ketefian's (1981) finding of a positive relationship between moral reasoning and moral behavior. The discrepancy in the findings may be interpreted as suggesting that the relationship between moral reasoning and moral behavior was complex and that other variables may have affected this relationship. Omery's findings (1986) regarding modes of reasoning and mitigating factors lent some support to this interpretation.

In his extensive review of literature related to moral action, Blasi (1980) reported that moral reasoning and moral action are related, depending on the outcome criteria used. For example, his findings gave evidence that individuals at higher reasoning stages tended to be more honest than those at lower stages, but there was no evidence to indicate that higher-stage thinkers were more likely to resist pressure to conform in their moral actions. In a similar vein, Rest (1983) suggested that moral reasoning is one of four components required to produce moral behavior. These components were cited as follows: (a) the person needs to have "moral sensitivity" and recognize the moral possibilities in a situation and the consequences of different courses of action on the welfare of others; (b) the person needs to make a judgment about the moral course of action; (c) the person needs to have "moral motivation," to place morality above other competing considerations; and (d) the person needs to have "moral character," and have sufficient persistence and know-how of implementation strategies to actually carry out the behavior (Schlaefli, Rest, & Thoma, 1985).

A tentative pattern was suggested, that selected organizational and work environment variables may predict some aspects of ethical practice. Measurement limitations possibly may have obscured the relationship between these work environment variables and ethical practice. As noted earlier, the specific dependent variables studied were quite different, and many of the investigator-constructed measures lacked support for reliability and validity.

There was little evidence that the research summarized here is cumulative, with each study building on preceding ones. Investigators have not learned from preceding research, nor have they built on the work of predecessors in any direct way. Knowledge accrual and theory building can occur only when research efforts are planned systematically (Ketefian, 1987).

There were no replications of studies in the group reviewed, nor did it seem that any of these studies replicated those conducted prior to 1983. However, in a few instances a specific finding in a study in effect did replicate a specific aspect of another study. Such instances provided the bases for drawing some conclusions in this review.

On the whole, studies tend to be too focused on the qualities of nurses; examination of environmental and organizational variables seemed to yield fruitful results, but these comprise a small proportion of the total studies reviewed. It is also worthwhile to investigate the interactions between person-related variables and factors that relate to the environment and work setting.

Most researchers have examined the effect of one or two selected variables on either moral reasoning or ethical practice. Yet by their nature these phenomena are so complex that multivariate research strategies and multiple measures can explain these phenomena more effectively. A case in point relates to efforts to explain ethical practice from the moral reasoning of subjects. A significant trend indicating a relationship has not emerged in these studies, possibly because moral reasoning is one of many components required to produce moral behavior.

A number of unanswered questions and future research directions that might be productive have been suggested in this review. These recommendations are identified below.

1. *Definition and measurement of ethical practice.* This construct and relevant elements need conceptual clarity. Investigators need to use the same nomenclature to refer to the phenomenon. The phenomenon of interest is nurses' ethical practice, which can be viewed meaningfully as an aspect of the overall practice of professional nursing rather than as an isolated entity.

Even more urgent attention needs to be directed to measurement. Without valid and reliable measures the knowledge yield is questionable at best. The profession as a whole has demonstrated greater appreciation of the importance of measurement of phenomena as a valuable research endeavor and goal in and of itself, deserving of full attention. However, the studies reviewed here reflect scant attention to measures.

Faculty in doctoral programs should encourage tool development as an acceptable topic for dissertation research. This matter is one of special interest, given that 28 of the 34 studies reviewed in this essay were dissertations, suggesting that much of the research in this area is being conducted by doctoral students.

2. *Predictors of ethical practice.* A large body of literature on professional practice within organizations suggests that there are inherent features in institutional practices, structures, rules, and regulations that pose important constraints to professional and hence ethical practice. Yet much research has been focused on the nurse and nurse characteristics as determinants of ethical practice. This focus on the nurse is a shortsighted view and leaves out important barriers that constrain nurses. Given that a large part of nursing practice occurs in organizational settings, investigators need to study how institutional policies, rules, and practices constrain ethical practice, and indeed, ways in which these factors create ethical dilemmas.

3. *Current ethical dilemmas.* Recent advances in science and technological developments in health care have created new ethical dilemmas for health professionals. There are an increasing number of governmental, professional, and institutional policies, rules, and regulations intended to regulate practices in regard to such matters. Examples of these relate to definition of death, determination of standards of patient competence, and issues related to informed consent and its implementation. There are numerous value judgments that professionals must make and ethical issues that they must confront frequently in their practice. Empirical studies of research questions that emanate from these areas could be of great benefit to patients, nurses, and others.

4. *Study design and measurement.* More rigorous study designs and measurement would strengthen this area of research and enhance confidence in the findings. Investigators needed to pay careful attention to the conceptual underpinnings on which instruments were based, use them appropriately, and adhere to established canons of scientific research design. For instance, there were a number of instances in which tests were modified, but the original reliability and validity were assumed to remain. In cases of quasi-experimental design, groups were not equivalent; given this fact, no pretest measures were obtained to control for preexisting group differences. In some cases pretest measures were available; yet these were not utilized in analyses to control for preexisting differences.

5. *Team research.* Team research needs to be encouraged in the field. In order to build programmatic research that is designed to

approach knowledge accrual systematically and over time, teamwork is necessary. In addition, such an approach will make it feasible to design complex studies using multiple measures and multivariate designs.

6. *Publication of research reports.* Only 3 of the 28 dissertations reviewed were published, one in a nursing research journal and two in nursing specialty journals. The low rate of publication is regrettable in view of the general inaccessibility and cost of obtaining dissertations. It is recommended that mentors urge nurses completing dissertations to report their research in the literature for wider dissemination.

7. *Replication.* The value of replication research has been discussed in the nursing literature and needs to be reiterated in this context as well. Replications increase confidence in research findings and prevent unwarranted implementation of significant results that may have been due to chance.

8. *Theoretical considerations.* In recent years there has evolved a different conception of women's development, morality, and, indeed, their views of the world as distinctive. Gilligan's (1982) challenge of Kohlberg's view of morality can be viewed within the broader context of the feminist literature. In a profession that is predominantly female, serious attention needs to be given to these alternative perspectives. Nurse investigators should incorporate these conceptions in the theoretical underpinnings of their studies, as well as be attentive to measures that embody these conceptions.

REFERENCES

Akerlund, B. M., & Norberg, A. (1985). An ethical analysis of double bind conflicts as experienced by care workers feeding severely demented patients. *International Journal of Nursing Studies, 22,* 207–216.

American Nurses' Association. (1976). *Code for nurses with interpretive statements.* Kansas City, MO: Author.

———. (1985). *Code for nurses with interpretive statements.* Kansas City, MO: Author.

Aronovitz, F. B. (1984). Autonomy, socialization, strength of religious belief and socioeconomic status as predictors of moral judgment in associate degree nursing students (Doctoral dissertation, University of Miami, 1984). *Dissertation Abstracts International, 46,* 112B.

Beardslee, N. Q. (1983). Survey of teaching ethics in nursing programs and the investigation of the relationship between extent of ethics content and moral reasoning levels (Doctoral dissertation, University of Northern Colorado, 1983). *Dissertation Abstracts International, 44,* 2380B.

Bell, C. M. W. (1983). Adult life crises, sexism, and moral reasoning in female nurses (Doctoral dissertation, Texas Woman's University, 1983). *Dissertation Abstracts International, 45,* 126B.

Bell, S. K. (1984). Effect of a biomedical ethics course on senior nursing students' level of moral development (Doctoral dissertation, West Virginia University, 1984). *Dissertation Abstracts International, 45,* 3205B.

Blasi, A. (1980). Bridging moral cognition and moral action: A critical review of the literature. *Psychological Bulletin, 88,* 1–45.

Bode, J., & Page, R. (1978). Comparison of measures of moral judgment. *Psychological Reports, 43,* 307–312.

Brown, P. I. (1974). Moral judgment and helpfulness toward a former mental patient (Doctoral dissertation, University of Texas at Austin, 1974). *Dissertation Abstracts International, 35,* 2399B–2400B.

Colby, A., Kohlberg, L., Gibbs, J., Candee, D., Speicher-Dubin, B., & Hewer, A. (1983). *The measurement of moral judgment: Standard issue scoring manuals.* Cambridge, MA: Harvard University, Center for Moral Development and Education.

Colby, A., Kohlberg, L., Gibbs, J., & Lieberman, M. (1983). A longitudinal study of moral judgment. *Monographs of the Society for Research in Child Development, 48*(1–2), Serial No. 200.

Cooper, H. M. (1982). Scientific guidelines for conducting integrative research reviews. *Review of Educational Research, 52,* 291–302.

Copstead, L. C. (1983). An examination of relationships: Perceived normative ethical stance/perceived realistic ethical choice and self-esteem among selected groups of registered nurses in Washington State (Doctoral dissertation, Gonzaga University, 1983). *Dissertation Abstracts International, 45,* 84A.

Cox, J. L. (1986). Ethical decision making by hospital nurses (Doctoral dissertation, Wayne State University, 1985). *Dissertation Abstracts International, 47,* 131B.

Crisham, P. (1981). Measuring moral judgment in nursing dilemmas. *Nursing Research, 30,* 104–110.

Curtin, L. L. (1978). Nursing ethics: Theories and pragmatics. *Nursing Forum, 17,* 4–11.

Davidson, M. L., & Robbins, S. (1978). The reliability and validity of objective indices of moral development. *Applied Psychological Measurement, 2,* 391–403.

de Jong, A. F. (1985). The relationship of moral reasoning and perceived autonomy at work to ethical judgment among female registered nurses (Doctoral dissertation, New York University, 1984). *Dissertation Abstracts International, 46,* 792B.

Dewey, J. (1964). What psychology can do for the teacher. In D. R. Archambault (Ed.), *John Dewey on education: Selected writings* (pp. 195–211). New York: Random House.

Dison, N. J. (1986). Dilemmas of baccalaureate nursing students (Doctoral dissertation, University of Minnesota, 1985). *Dissertation Abstracts International, 46,* 3390B.

Epstein, J. (1978). Moral judgment and positive concern for others and responsibility in conduct (Doctoral dissertation, New York University, 1977). *Dissertation Abstracts International, 38,* 6235B–6236B.

Felton, G. M. (1984). Attribution of responsibility, ethical/moral reasoning and the ability of undergraduate and graduate nursing students to resolve ethical/moral dilemmas (Doctoral dissertation, University of South Carolina, 1984). *Dissertation Abstracts International, 46,* 474B.

Felton, G. M., & Parsons, M. A. (1987). The impact of nursing education on ethical/moral decision making. *Journal of Nursing Education, 26,* 7–11.

Finch, A. J. (1986). Relationship between organizational climate and nurses' ethical decisions (Doctoral dissertation, University of Texas at Austin, 1986). *Dissertation Abstracts International, 47,* 1927B.

Fleeger, R. L. (1986). Critical thinking and moral reasoning behavior of baccalaureate nursing students (Doctoral dissertation, Claremont Graduate School, 1986). *Dissertation Abstracts International, 47,* 1915B.

Forman, E. C. (1986). Professional nurses' level of moral reasoning and attitudes toward mental illness (Doctoral dissertation, University of Houston, 1986). *Dissertation Abstracts International, 47,* 2898A.

Frisch, N. C. (1986). The value analysis model and the moral and cognitive development of baccalaureate nursing students (Doctoral dissertation, Southern Illinois University at Carbondale, 1986). *Dissertation Abstracts International, 47,* 2467A.

Ganong, L. H. (1987). Integrative reviews of nursing research. *Research in Nursing and Health, 10,* 1–11.

Garritson, S. H. (1986). The influence of psychiatric inpatient environments on ethical decision making of psychiatric nurses (Doctoral dissertation, University of California at San Francisco, 1985). *Dissertation Abstracts International, 46,* 2622B.

Gaul, A. L. (1987a). The effect of a course in nursing ethics on the relationship between ethical choice and ethical action in baccalaureate nursing students. *Journal of Nursing Education, 26,* 113–117.

Gaul, A. L. (1987b). Moral reasoning and ethical decision making in nursing practice (Doctoral dissertation, Texas Woman's University, 1986). *Dissertation Abstracts International, 47,* 4113B.

Gilligan, C. (1982). *In a different voice.* Cambridge, MA: Harvard University Press.

Gortner, S. R. (1985). Ethical inquiry. *Annual Review of Nursing Research, 3,* 193–214.

Holly, C. M. (1986). Staff nurses' participation in ethical decision making: A descriptive study of selected situational variables (Doctoral dissertation, Teachers College, Columbia University, 1986). *Dissertation Abstracts International, 47,* 2372B.

Holzman, P. G. (1984). A comparative study of liberal arts and nursing students' moral development in collegiate programs (Doctoral dissertation, Marquette University, 1984). *Dissertation Abstracts International, 45,* 3772B.

Husted, G. L. (1983). Testing an ethical decision-making model for nurses (Doctoral dissertation, University of Pittsburgh, 1983). *Dissertation Abstracts International, 45,* 513B.

Jackson, G. B. (1980). Methods for integrative reviews. *Review of Educational Research, 50,* 438–460.

Jacobs, M. K. (1977). The DIT related to behavior in an experimental setting: Promise keeping in the Prisoner's Dilemma Game. In J. R. Rest, J. Carroll, J. Lawrence, K. Jacobs, E. McColgan, M. Davidson, & S. Robbins (Eds.), *Development in judging moral issues* (Technical Report No. 3, pp. 48–59). Minneapolis: Minnesota Moral Research Projects.

Jameton, A. (1977). The nurse: When rules and roles conflict. *Hastings Center Report, 7*(4), 22–23.

Kay, S. R. (1982). Kohlberg's theory of moral development: Critical analysis of validation studies with the defining issues test. *International Journal of Psychology, 17,* 27–42.

Keller, M. C. (1985). Nurses' responses to moral dilemmas (Doctoral dissertation, University of South Carolina, 1985). *Dissertation Abstracts International, 46,* 1870B.

Kellmer, D. M. (1984). The teaching of ethical decision making in schools of nursing: Variables and strategies (Doctoral dissertation, Gonzaga University, 1984). *Dissertation Abstracts International, 45,* 1732B.

Ketefian, S. (1981). Moral reasoning and moral behavior among selected groups of practicing nurses. *Nursing Research, 30,* 171–176.

Ketefian, S. (1982). Tool development in nursing: Construction of a scale to measure moral behavior. *The Journal of the New York State Nurses' Association, 13*(2), 13–18.

Ketefian, S. (1984). *Measuring moral behavior in nursing: Research strategy in tool development.* Unpublished manuscript, University of Michigan, Ann Arbor.

Ketefian, S. (1985). Professional and bureaucratic role conceptions and moral behavior among nurses. *Nursing Research, 34,* 248–253.

Ketefian, S. (1987). A case study of theory development: Moral behavior in nursing. *Advances in Nursing Science, 9*(2), 10–19.

Kohlberg, L. (1971). From is to ought: How to commit the naturalistic fallacy and get away with it in the study of moral development. In T. Mitschel (Ed.), *Cognitive development and epistemology* (pp. 151–235). New York: Academic Press.

Kohlberg, L. (1978). The cognitive-developmental approach to moral education. In P. Scharf (Ed.), *Readings in moral education* (pp. 36–51). Minneapolis, MN: Winston Press.

Kohlberg, L., Levine, C., & Hewer, A. (1984). Moral stages: A current statement. Response to critics. Appendix A. In L. Kohlberg (Ed.), *The psychology of moral development* (pp. 207–386, 621–639). *Essays on Moral Development* (Vol. 2). New York: Harper & Row.

Lawrence, J., & Crisham, P. (1984). A study in resolutions. *Nursing Times, 80*(30), 53–55.

Mayberry, M. A. (1983). Moral reasoning in ethical dilemmas of staff nurses and head nurses (Doctoral dissertation, University of Southern California, 1983). *Dissertation Abstracts International, 44,* 2240A.

Mayberry, M. A. (1986). Ethical decision making: A response of hospital nurses. *Nursing Administration Quarterly, 10*(3), 75–81.

McNamee, S. (1978). Moral behavior, moral development and motivation. *Journal of Moral Education, 7,* 27–32.

Munhall, P. L. (1980). Moral reasoning levels of nursing students and faculty in a baccalaureate nursing program. *Image, 12,* 57–61.

Murphy, C. C. (1977). Levels of moral reasoning in a selected group of nursing practitioners (Doctoral dissertation, Teachers College, Columbia University, 1976). *Dissertation Abstracts International, 38,* 593B–594B.

Mustapha, S. L. W. (1985). An examination of moral reasoning in college students in two types of education curricula: Implications for nursing education (Doctoral dissertation, University of Kansas, 1985). *Dissertation Abstracts International, 47,* 428A.

Nokes, K. M. (1985). The relationship between moral reasoning, the relationship dimension of the social climate of the work environment, and perception of realistic moral behavior among registered professional nurses (Doctoral dissertation, New York University, 1986). *Dissertation Abstracts International, 46,* 1119B.

Omery, A. K. (1986). The moral reasoning of nurses who work in the adult intensive care setting (Doctoral dissertation, Boston University, 1985). *Dissertation Abstracts International, 46,* 3007B.

Ott, B. B. (1986). An ethical problem facing nurses: The support of patient autonomy in the do not resuscitate decision (Doctoral dissertation, Texas Woman's University, 1986). *Dissertation Abstracts International, 47,* 1930B.

Pence, T. (1986). *Ethics in nursing: An annotated bibliography* (Pub. No. 20-1989). New York: National League for Nursing.

Piaget, J. (1965). *The moral judgment of the child.* New York: The Free Press. (Originally published 1932)

Pinch, W. J. (1985). Ethical dilemmas in nursing: The role of the nurse and perceptions of autonomy. *Journal of Nursing Education, 24,* 372–376.

Rest, J. (1974a). Developmental psychology as a guide to value education: A review of "Kohlbergian" programs. *Review of Educational Research, 44,* 241–259.

Rest, J. (1974b). *Manual for the Defining Issues Test.* Minneapolis: The University of Minnesota.

Rest, J. (1975a). Longitudinal study of the Defining Issues Test of moral judgment: A strategy for analyzing developmental change. *Developmental Psychology, 11,* 738–748.

Rest, J. (1975b). Recent research in an objective test of moral judgment. In D. J. DePalma & J. M. Foley (Eds.), *Moral development: Current theory and research.* New York: Wiley.

Rest, J. (1976). New approaches in the assessment of moral judgment. In T. Lickona (Ed.), *Moral development and behavior: Theory, research and social issues* (pp. 198–218). New York: Holt, Rinehart and Winston.

Rest, J. (1979). *Development in judging moral issues.* Minneapolis: University of Minnesota Press.

Rest, J. (1983). Morality. In J. Flavell & E. Markman (Eds.), *Cognitive development* (Vol. 3, 4th Ed., pp. 556–629). In P. Mussen (General Ed.), *Handbook of child psychology.* New York: Wiley.

Rest, J., Turiel, E., & Kohlberg, L. (1969). Levels of moral development as a determinant of preference and comprehension of moral judgments made by others. *Journal of Personality, 37,* 225–252.

Schlaefli, A., Rest, J. J., & Thoma, S. J. (1985). Does moral education improve moral judgment? A meta-analysis of intervention studies using the Defining Issues Test. *Review of Educational Research, 55,* 319–352.

Staub, E. (1974). Helping a distressed person: Social, personality, and stimulus determinants. In L. Berkowitz (Ed.), *Advances in experimental social psychology* (pp. 301–329). New York: Academic Press.

Subject guide to books in print 1985–1986 (Vol. 3). (1985). New York: R. R. Bowker Co.

Swider, S. M., McElmurry, B. J., & Yarling, R. R. (1985). Ethical decision making in a bureaucratic context by senior nursing students. *Nursing Research, 34,* 108–112.

Turner, V. A. (1984). The relationship between moral judgment and moral action among professional nurses (Doctoral dissertation, Fordham University, 1984). *Dissertation Abstracts International, 45,* 2026A.

Winland-Brown, J. E. (1983). A comparison of student nurses, nurses and non-nurses with regard to their moral judgments on nursing dilemmas (Doctoral dissertation, Florida Atlantic University, 1983). *Dissertation Abstracts International, 44,* 336B.

Zablow, R. J. (1985). Preparing students for the moral dimension of professional nursing practice: A protocol for nurse educators (Doctoral dissertation, Teachers College, Columbia University, 1984). *Dissertation Abstracts International, 45,* 2501B.

PART V

Other Research

Chapter 10

Patient Education: Part II

CAROL A. LINDEMAN
SCHOOL OF NURSING
THE OREGON HEALTH SCIENCES UNIVERSITY

CONTENTS

This review is the second of two chapters in which published nursing research on patient education is summarized and inferences drawn for a theory of instruction for patient education. The first chapter, in Volume 6 of the *Annual Review of Nursing Research* (Lindeman, 1988), included research related to the following five categories of variables: (a) characteristics of the patient as learner; (b) characteristics of the nurse as teacher; (c) nurse–patient interaction as instructional strategy; (d) characteristics of the target group; and (e) the health care setting as the learning environment. This review includes research in which the content of the patient education intervention was the primary variable.

To identify studies for the review, computerized searches using MEDLINE and the Educational Resources Information Center (ERIC) were done with the following subtitles: patient education, comparative

199

studies, clinical trials, evaluation studies, and preoperative education. The *International Nursing Index* and *Cumulative Index to Nursing and Allied Health Literature* were hand-searched for the years 1965 to 1986, and the bibliographies of all retrieved articles were examined for potential studies for this review. Those articles having a nurse as the first author and reporting adequate information about every phase of the research process were included in the total data base of 120 articles. Of the 29 studies meeting the criteria for inclusion in this part of the review, 9 were centered on systematic relaxation or biofeedback as content, 14 were designed using a psychoeducational intervention, and 6 were focused on parenting behaviors. These three areas of content serve as the organizing framework for this chapter.

RELAXATION AND BIOFEEDBACK AS CONTENT

Among the studies identified for this review, nine included exploration of systematic relaxation and biofeedback as content for patient education programs. Of the seven studies in which the patient education content was systematic relaxation, one investigator used a single-group design and six used control-group designs. In the two studies in which the content was biofeedback, one investigator used a single-group design and one used a control-group design.

Cotanch (1983) described the effectiveness of progressive muscle relaxation (PMR) in reducing nausea and vomiting and anxiety in a group of 12 cancer patients. The patients were experiencing refractory drug-induced nausea and vomiting and served as their own controls. The investigator gave the subjects personal instruction in PMR, presenting it as a skill that needed to be learned through practice. They were to view PMR as a self-control technique that they could choose whether or not to use. Data were analyzed by measuring a straight percentage change from baseline to subsequent time periods. Nausea and vomiting were improved in 9 of the 12 subjects 48 hours postchemotherapy. All subjects improved their caloric intake during that same time frame. All patients reported that the relaxation technique made them feel more comfortable and in control.

The six investigators using control-group designs studied the effects of relaxation training on dependent variables associated with pain and tension. Bafford (1976) reported that the subjects receiving instruction in relaxation did not differ significantly on measures of pain, distress, and mental disturbance from subjects visited but not instructed and subjects neither visited nor instructed. Flaherty and Fitzpatrick (1978) found significant differences on measures of pain, distress, and respiration between postoperative patients instructed in a relaxation technique and those subjects not instructed. Wells (1982) also used surgical subjects and reported that subjects receiving relaxation training had lower distress scores than subjects receiving general preoperative instruction. The groups did not differ on measures of muscle tension, intensity of pain, or analgesic use. Tamez, Moore, and Brown (1978) conducted their research with psychiatric patients receiving minor tranquilizers and minor sedatives. Their primary hypothesis that relaxation training would reduce the frequency of intake of pro re nata medications was not supported.

Two investigators using control-group designs investigated the effects of relaxation training on psychological variables. Aiken and Henrichs (1971) analyzed the effects of relaxation training on postoperative psychiatric reactions with open-heart surgery patients. There was a trend toward fewer complications in the group receiving relaxation instruction in comparison with the control group. Bohachick (1984) also reported significant positive effects on anxiety and selected psychological symptoms with subjects in a cardiac exercise program who received relaxation training when compared to subjects not receiving the instruction.

The two studies in which investigators explored the effects of biofeedback showed beneficial effects. Janson-Bjerklie and Clarke (1982) found significant differences in control of bronchial diameter between subjects receiving biofeedback and those subjects receiving random feedback. Sitzman, Kamiya, and Johnston (1983) used a single-group design and reported descriptive data supporting positive effects on breathing patterns from using techniques of biofeedback training.

Although these studies were focused on the same independent variable at the conceptual level, at an operational level the content of the instructional sessions differed. For example, Cotanch (1983) taught progressive muscle relaxation as a skill and a self-control technique. Flaherty and Fitzpatrick (1978) taught a relaxation technique of letting the lower jaw drop slightly and keeping the tongue quiet. In addition, the number of teaching sessions varied from study to study. In most studies the investigator was the patient instructor and data collector. Investigators also reported difficulty with the measurement of dependent variables associated with pain and distress. Bafford (1976), for example, had difficulty in interpreting data as a result of postoperative complications and differences in preoperative health status.

Despite the conceptual and methodological limitations presented by this group of studies, overall the results are promising. It would appear that relaxation training and biofeedback are content areas for which patient education results in measurable benefits for the patients instructed.

PSYCHOEDUCATIONAL CONTENT

There were 14 studies in the data base in which investigators conceptualized the hospital illness experience as a threatening event and the experimental intervention as primarily psychological and secondarily educational. The studies are reported in chronological order with the exception of the Johnson studies, which are presented in sequence.

Dumas and Leonard (1963) reported a three-phase study in which they explored the effect of an experimental nursing approach on postoperative vomiting. The experimental nursing approach was a process of nursing directed toward helping the patient achieve a suitable psychological state for surgery. The process involved (a) an exploration of patient behavior to determine the presence or absence of experienced distress and an exploration of the cause of distress and approaches needed to relieve the distress; (b) a determination of appropriate actions to relieve the distress; and (c) an evaluation of outcomes. Data analysis for the combined subjects from all three phases showed a significant decrease in vomiting for the experimental subjects in comparison with subjects not receiving the experimental approach.

Meyers (1964) explored the effects of three methods of communication on patients' responses to an unfamiliar and moderately stressful situation. A total of 72 patients was assigned to one of three groups: structured communication explaining the situation, no communication, and distracting/irrelevant communication. After the event, data on subjects' feelings and recall were collected through interview. Analysis of the responses from the interview provided five scores: an accuracy score, a blood-needle score, an overestimation score, an underestimation score, and a talkativeness score. A chi-square test was applied to the frequency data for each dependent variable. The data led the investigator to conclude that giving the patient structured information decreased tension and added to comfort, and distracting the patient was stressful.

Elms and Leonard (1966) compared the effects of three admission procedures on stress. A total of 75 patients were assigned according to block randomization to one of three admission procedure groups. One group received an individualized approach that was focused on the patient. A second group received an approach that was focused on the procedure. In this approach the patient was supplied with information about the hospital, but no effort was made to respond to individual needs for information or support. The third group received routine care. There were no significant differences in patient satisfaction, temperature, or blood pressure. Subjects in the individualized approach group had lower pulse and respiration rates.

Schmitt and Wooldridge (1973) investigated the effects of a group discussion for preoperative patients on postoperative recovery. The group discussion provided an opportunity for patients to discuss fears and to receive information. An experimental design was used with 25 subjects in each of the two groups. Subjects were matched in terms of surgical procedure and did not differ in terms of age, occupation, job status, or religious preference. Although experimental patients did use less pain medication, resumed an oral diet sooner, and required less anesthesia and a shorter induction time, the differences were not statistically significant. The investigators concluded from use of clinical and statistical data that the experimental nursing intervention did reduce stress.

Langer, Janis, and Wolfer (1975) compared a coping device strategy with preparatory information using 60 surgical patients. The coping device entailed the cognitive reappraisal of anxiety-provoking events, calming self-talk, and cognitive control through selective attention. Dependent variables included pre- and postoperative stress, analgesics, and sedatives. Pre- and postoperative stress were assessed by obtaining ratings from nurses on the wards. Nurses were asked to rate level of anxiety and degree of dealing with anxiety. The total number of pain relievers and sedatives were taken from the record. In addition, blood pressure and pulse readings were recorded before and 15 minutes after the interview and again before and about 1 hour after the operation. A significant effect from the coping device strategy was shown on these dependent variables.

Seven studies by Johnson and colleagues have been included in this review. They represented a systematic evaluation of a consistent psychoeducational strategy. Johnson (1972) described the early development and testing in the laboratory and clinical setting of the hypothesis that accurate expectations about sensations reduce stress. Johnson and Leventhal (1974) reported an experiment in which the subjects were 48 hospitalized patients receiving an endoscopic examination. The research design included four treatment groups: sensory description information, behavioral information, sensory behavioral combination, and no preparatory information. The sensory description information included what would be done to the patient and the specific sensations he would experience during the examination. The behavioral instructions included specific instructions for rapid mouth breathing and panting and actions to take while the tube was being inserted. The instructions were tape-recorded. Dependent variables were classed as indicators of emotional reactions and indicators of performance. The behavioral measures used to assess these variables were milligrams of tranquilizer required for sedation, heart rate changes during the examinations, hand and arm movements during tube passage, and number of seconds required to pass the tube into the stomach. For the behavioral instruction group, there was a reduction in the dosage of tranquilizer, a stabilization of heart rate, and a slight reduction in number of patients observed gagging, but none of these comparisons with the control group were significant. Patients in the sensory description group received significantly fewer milligrams of tranquilizers and had more stable heart rates than controls for patients under 50 years of age. Also, gagging was reduced significantly. Patients in the combined condition showed more stable heart rates for subjects under 50, marked reductions in gagging, and an increase in time for tube passage. Interpretation of these findings led the investigators to conclude that specific types of information could be used to reduce aversive responses and to strengthen effective coping responses.

Using this same basic theoretical framework and design, Johnson reported the following series of experiments. Johnson, Kirchhoff, and Endress (1975) investigated the use of sensory and behavioral preparatory information to reduce the distress of children having orthopedic casts removed. As in the previous study (Johnson & Leventhal, 1974), the sensation group received instruction regarding the procedure for cast removal and the sensations that would be experienced. The procedure group received detailed information about the procedure for cast removal. The mean distress score for the sensation group differed significantly from the control group. The procedure information group did not differ significantly from the controls. Fuller, Endress, and Johnson (1978) reported on the use of cognitive and behavioral information on women undergoing pelvic and breast examinations. The results of the study supported the effect of preparatory sensory information on stress reduction associated with an aversive event.

Johnson, Rice, Fuller, and Endress (1978) reported on the use of various preparatory messages on two groups of surgical patients: cholecystectomy and herniorrhaphy. In the first study with cholecystectomy subjects, the positive effect of the sensory information message seen in previous studies was demonstrated. A 2×3 experimental factorial design was used with instruction and information as experimental factors. Instruction consisted of detailed step-by-step instruction on deep breathing, coughing, and bed exercises. Instruction consisted of procedure information and/or sensation information. In the second study with subjects undergoing herniorrhaphy, a positive effect was not observed. The same investigators reported a replication of their work (Johnson, Fuller, Endress, & Rice, 1978), modifying the design to include analysis of effects from prehospital admission preparation, restatement of preparatory information postoperatively, and the addition of temporal orienting information. A sample of 58 cholecystectomy and 57 herniorrhaphy patients were assigned randomly to one of five treatment groups. The main effects of the earlier studies were replicated. Sensory information was found to be most effective when combined with instruction in postoperative exercises. The preparatory interventions had no significant effects on the indicators of rate of recovery for the herniorrhaphy patients.

Johnson, Christman, and Stitt (1985) conducted a 2-phase study to evaluate the short- and long-term effects of various types of preparatory information. The sample consisted of 168 hysterectomy patients who were divided randomly into groups to receive the intervention: cognitive coping technique information, behavioral concrete sensory information, or the usual care control condition. Concrete sensory information was expected to increase patients' confidence in existing coping abilities, foster versatility in use of coping strategies, and lead to an early resumption of usual life activities. The instruction in this study was methods of moving and getting out of bed to minimize discomfort. Data were collected during hospitalization and 1, 4, and 12 weeks after discharge. Patients were assigned randomly to experimental discharge information or control discharge information groups. Measured were pain, discomfort, mood states, and physical recovery. Patients were interviewed as to coping techniques and process used during hospitalization. Hospital charts were used to obtain information on postoperative complications, anesthesia, medication use, and length of hospitalization. Results indicated that the behavioral coping technique patients reduced the amount of pain medication used, whereas the cognitive coping technique patients reported better physical recovery during hospitalization, but a longer hospitalization. There was much missing data in the posthospitalization measurements. Overall, 70% of the patients returned the data sets for all three occasions of measurement after discharge; but this return represented 81% of the control discharge group and 58% of the experimental discharge group. Ninety-four percent of the patients who received the behavioral coping instructions reported they used it in ambulating, whereas 17% who received cognitive coping instructions reported they used it. The hypotheses were not supported to the extent the investigators anticipated.

Hartfield and Cason (1981) extended Johnson's work by controlling for anxiety proneness. The subjects were 24 hospitalized patients receiving a barium enema. They were assigned randomly to one of three groups: sensation information, procedure information, or control group. Data were collected before the information, after the information, and after the procedure. The Spielberger, Gorsuch, and Lushene (1970) Trait Anxiety Inventory was used as a measure of behavioral disposition, and State Anxiety Inventory (Fuller, Endress, & Johnson, 1978; Johnson, Kirchhoff, & Endress, 1975) was used as a measure of emotional response. The significant difference between mean anxiety scores of the sensation and the procedure groups in the absence of a significant difference between mean anxiety scores of the sensation and no information groups in this study varied from the previous reports of Johnson and others. The postinformation data showed that the sensation group had significantly less anxiety and more congruent expectations than the other.

Hill (1982) used the Johnson framework in an experimental design with 40 cataract patients as subjects. Subjects were assigned randomly to behavioral instructions, sensory information, both behavioral and sensory information, or general information. Dependent variables included postoperative mood state and length of recovery time. There were no significant differences between groups on any of the dependent measures, with one exception. The combination of sensory and behavioral information group reported significantly fewer number of days after discharge before venturing out of the house.

This series of studies can be viewed as rather distinctive in this phase of the development of the discipline of nursing. The research has a strong theory and practice base. Early investigations laid the groundwork for the theoretical formulations made explicit by Johnson and Leventhal (1974). Johnson individually and then with colleagues systematically tested the theory and its generalizability. This systematic evaluation of practice-relevant theory is a model that deserves recognition.

The psychoeducational interventions appear relatively powerful for a range of subjects. The failure to produce equally positive outcomes with some subjects suggests that important variables, possibly interacting with the instructional intervention, have yet to be isolated. The relationship of this intervention to a more traditional educational intervention also needs to be explored in terms of other factors relevant to a theory of instruction, for example, patient characteristics.

PARENTING BEHAVIORS

Six investigators reported studies on the effectiveness of patient education and subsequent behavior of the mother or father toward the infant. Hall (1980) conducted an experimental study to determine the effect of a structured, informative, in-home nursing intervention. The sample of 30 postpartum mothers was assigned randomly to either the experimental group or a control group. The control group received no home instruction. The dependent variable was the mother's perception of the infant as measured by the Neonatal Perception Inventories I and II (Broussard, 1965). Data analysis supported a significant positive change for the experimental but not the control group.

Bowen and Miller (1980) conducted an exploratory study to determine the relationship between the father's attendance at parenthood classes, presence during delivery, and the state of the infant. A sample of 48 fathers was used. All fathers who met the criteria were asked to participate in the study. The fathers were divided into three groups: those who took classes and were present at delivery, those who did not take classes but were present at delivery, and those who did neither. Data analysis showed that attendance at delivery was associated significantly with demonstrating attachment behaviors; attendance at preparenthood classes was not.

Anderson (1981) used a sample of 30 primiparous mothers to compare the effects of two interventions designed to familiarize mothers with the individual capabilities and characteristics of their infants.

Mothers were assigned randomly to one of three groups: show-and-tell, tell-only, or information on infant furnishings. Maternal responsiveness, the dependent variable, was enhanced significantly in the show-and-tell group only.

Croft (1982) used an exploratory approach to evaluate the relationship between Lamaze childbirth education and maternal–infant attachment. A sample of 61 primiparous women was used; 45 had participated in Lamaze classes, and 16 had no prenatal preparation. Analysis of the data showed no significant differences in maternal attachment at one day postpartum; at one month postpartum the Lamaze mothers showed significantly lower degrees of attachment.

Perry (1983) evaluated the effects of a structured interaction of parent and infant on parents' perception of the infant. Parents were randomly assigned to one of four treatment groups: mother only, father only, both parents, no teaching. Data were collected using the Neonatal Perception Inventories I, II, and III (Broussard, 1965) and the Mother's Assessment of the Behavior of Her Infant (Field, Dempsey, Hallock, & Shuman, 1978). The investigator found no relationship between infant behavior and parental perception.

Riesch and Munns (1984) reported an experimental study on the effects of an educative nursing intervention with full-term mothers and its replication with preterm mothers. The dependent variable was the observations and responses of the mother. Data analysis showed that the treatment groups had significantly higher scores on posttest measures of both neonatal cues and self-reported behaviors. In addition, the treatment group's reports were significantly more congruent with the nurse's observations.

At an abstract level all the studies in this category were explorations of the effects of teaching parenting behaviors on later child and parent behaviors. However, at the operational level the instructional content differed from study to study. In addition, the investigators reported varying degrees of success in controlling variables affecting the success of their interventions. Croft (1982), for example, spoke to subject characteristics that must be controlled to have equivalent study groups. She also spoke to the need to control for hospital practices when designing research. Problems in measurement also were addressed by these investigators. For example, Perry (1983) discussed the difficulty in the measures of actual behavior and perception of behavior. The validity of certain inventories also was questioned.

Intuition supports the position that instruction in parenting behavior leads to more effective parent–child interactions. The state of the art in measurement of parent–child interactions and the diversity in conceptions of appropriate content in parenting behavior detract from the ability to support intuition by empirical evidence.

GENERALIZATIONS FOR THEORY OF INSTRUCTION

A total of 29 studies in which investigators addressed three specific content areas were included in the data base. The following generalizations are offered:

1. Biofeedback and relaxation training are effective for a range of patient groups and can alter both physiological and psychological health status outcomes.
2. Psychoeducational content does impact health status outcomes other than knowledge. The interaction between that instructional content, characteristics of patient, and group characteristics is not yet clear.
3. Instruction in parenting behavior is likely to have a positive influence on the parent–child interaction. However, prescribing specific content and experiences is unclear from the research to date.

CONCLUSIONS AND FUTURE DIRECTIONS

This review of patient education research included 29 studies in three content areas. The intent was to analyze the research in terms of the instructional content and to draw inferences for a theory of instruction. The three content areas in this review, relaxation and biofeedback, psychoeducational process, and parenting behavior, represent very complex areas of instruction. Attitudes and behaviors were involved as well as knowledge, facts, and skills. In many instances these complex instructional interventions were implemented in abbreviated time tables. Yet the majority of the investigators reported promising or statistically significant positive effects from their interventions.

The introduction of prospective financing for health care and the resulting shortened length of hospital stay have increased the importance of patient teaching as a nursing intervention. In this regard, content areas that would be valuable from a nursing practice perspective include discharge teaching, safe and effective use of prescribed technology, and family caregiver techniques. The changing patterns of medical care expenditures for chronic illness and health conditions associated with lifestyle and aging influences also increase the importance of patient education as a nursing intervention. Content areas that are associated with changes in health care include self-care practices, illness prevention, health promotion, and stress reduction.

The ability to address the contribution of content as a category of factors in a theory of instruction will require future investigators to describe thoroughly the educational intervention at both the conceptual and empirical levels. Without rich description at both of these levels it is extremely difficult, if not impossible, to categorize, analyze, and synthesize studies.

REFERENCES

Aiken, L., & Henrichs, T. (1971). Systematic relaxation as a nursing intervention technique with open heart surgery patients. *Nursing Research, 20,* 212–217.

Anderson, C. (1981). Enhancing reciprocity between mother and neonate. *Nursing Research, 30,* 89–93.

Bafford, D. (1976). Progressive relaxation as a nursing intervention: A method of controlling pain for open-heart surgery patients. In M.V. Batey (Ed.), *Communicating nursing research* (Vol. 8, pp. 284–290). Boulder, CO: Western Interstate Commission for Higher Education (WICHE).

Bohachick, P. (1984). Progressive relaxation training in cardiac rehabilitation: Effect on psychologic variables. *Nursing Research, 33,* 283–287.

Bowen, S., & Miller, B. (1980). Paternal attachment behavior as related to presence at delivery and preparenthood classes: A pilot study. *Nursing Research, 29,* 307–311.

Broussard, E. R. (1965). *A study to determine the effectiveness of television as a means of providing anticipatory counseling to primiparae during the postpartum period.* Unpublished doctoral dissertation, University of Pittsburgh, Pittsburgh.

Cotanch, P. (1983). Relaxation training for control of nausea and vomiting in patients receiving chemotherapy. *Cancer Nursing, 6,* 277–283.

Croft, C. (1982). Lamaze childbirth education: Implications for maternal-infant attachment. *Journal of Obstetric, Gynecologic, and Neonatal Nursing, 11,* 333–336.

Dumas, R., & Leonard, R. (1963). The effect of nursing on the incidence of postoperative vomiting. *Nursing Research, 12,* 12–15.

Elms, R., & Leonard, R. (1966). Effects of nursing approaches during admission. *Nursing Research, 15,* 39–48.

Field, T. M., Dempsey, J. R., Hallock, N. H., & Shuman, H. H. (1978). The mother's assessment of the behavior of her infant. *Infant Behavior and Development, 1,* 156–167.

Flaherty, G., & Fitzpatrick, J. (1978). Relaxation technique to increase comfort level of postoperative patients: A preliminary study. *Nursing Research, 27,* 352–355.

Fuller, S., Endress, P., & Johnson, J. (1978). The effects of cognitive and behavioral control on coping with an aversive health examination. *Journal of Human Stress, 4,* 18–25.

Hall, L. (1980). Effect of teaching on primiparas' perceptions of their newborn. *Nursing Research, 29,* 317–322.

Hartfield, M., & Cason, C. (1981). Effect of information on emotional responses during barium enema. *Nursing Research, 30,* 151–155.

Hill, B. (1982). Sensory information, behavioral instructions and coping with sensory alteration surgery. *Nursing Research, 31,* 17–21.

Janson-Bjerklie, S., & Clarke, E. (1982). The effects of biofeedback training on bronchial diameter in asthma. *Heart & Lung, 11,* 200–207.

Johnson, J. (1972). Effects of structuring patients' expectations on their reactions to threatening events. *Nursing Research, 21,* 499–503.

Johnson, J., Christman, N., & Stitt, C. (1985). Personal control interventions: Short and long term effects on surgical patients. *Research in Nursing and Health, 8,* 131–145.

Johnson, J., Fuller, S., Endress, M., & Rice, V. (1978). Altering patients' responses to surgery: An extension and replication. *Research in Nursing and Health, 1,* 111–121.

Johnson, J., Kirchhoff, K. T., & Endress, M. (1975). Altering children's distress behavior during orthopedic cast removal. *Nursing Research, 24,* 404–410.

Johnson, J., & Leventhal, H. (1974). Effects of accurate expectations and behavioral instructions on reactions during a noxious medical examination. *Journal of Personality and Social Psychology, 29,* 710–718.

Johnson, J., Rice, V., Fuller, S., & Endress, M. (1978). Sensory information, instruction in a coping strategy, and recovery from surgery. *Research in Nursing and Health, 1,* 4–17.

Langer, E., Janis, I., & Wolfer, J. (1975). Reduction of psychological stress in surgical patients. *Journal of Experimental Social Psychology, 11,* 155–165.

Lindeman, C. A. (1988). Patient education. *Annual Review of Nursing Research, 6,* 29–60.

Meyers, M. (1964). The effect of types of communication on patients' reactions to stress. *Nursing Research, 13,* 126–131.

Perry, S. (1983). Parents' perceptions of their newborn following structured interactions. *Nursing Research, 32,* 208–212.

Riesch, S., & Munns, S. (1984). Promoting awareness: The mother and her baby. *Nursing Research, 33,* 271–276.

Schmitt, F., & Wooldridge, P. (1973). Psychological preparation of surgical patients. *Nursing Research, 22,* 108–116.

Sitzman, J., Kamiya, J., & Johnston, J. (1983). Biofeedback training for reduced respiratory rate in chronic obstructive pulmonary disease: A preliminary study. *Nursing Research, 32,* 218–223.

Spielberger, C. D., Gorsuch, R. L., & Lushene, R. (1970). *Manual for the State-Trait Anxiety Inventory.* Palo Alto, CA: Consulting Psychologists Press.

Tamez, E., Moore, M., & Brown, P. (1978). Relaxation training as a nursing intervention versus pro re nata medication. *Nursing Research, 27,* 160–164.

Wells, N. (1982). The effect of relaxation on postoperative muscle tension and pain. *Nursing Research, 31,* 236–238.

Index

Acquired immunodeficiency
  syndrome (AIDS), 99
Adelstein, W., 18, 23
Adikofer, Sr. R. M., 32, 46
Adolescent Identity Confusion, 136
Adult Respiratory Distress
  Syndrome (ARDS), 29
Age, and moral reasoning, 180–181
Aged, *See* Older persons
AIDS, infection control, 99
Aiken, L., 201, 210
Ainslie, B., 167, 169
Akerlund, B. M., 183, 185, 190
Akerstedt, T., 86, 92
Albert, R. K., 99, 110
Alexander, Cheryl S.:
  Parent-child nursing education,
  157–170
Allen, G. A., 121, 138
Alteration:
  in comfort; diagnosis of pain, 122
  in parenting; diagnosis, 122
*American Journal of Infection
  Control,* 96
American Nurses' Association, 161,
  182, 190
  definition of nursing, 117, 138
Amidon, D., 74, 76, 77, 92
Amoroso, R., 124, 127, 129, 140
Anders, T. T., 75, 80, 90
Andersen, L., 167, 169
Anderson, C., 207, 210
Angelopoulos, N., 84, 91
Antonovsky, K. A., 66
Anxiety, 61
  diagnosis, 121, 132
  patient education, 206

Anxiety-Depression Scale, 131
Apnea, 34–35, 87
  treatments, 87
Arkins, R. E., 31, 48
Aronovitz, F. B., 178, 179, 180,
  181, 190
Arterial oxygen levels, 32
Aseptic techniques, 102–103,
  105–106
Association for Practitioners in
  Infection Control (APIC), 96
Attire, and infection control,
  101–102
Avant, K., 134, 138
Awareness:
  altered levels; diagnosis, 132
Ayllon, T., 145, 152
Azrin, N. H., 145, 152

Baas, L. S., 121, 138
Babcock, H., 23
Babcock Story Recall, 15
Backman, M., 164, 169
Baekeland, F., 83, 90
Bafford, D., 200, 201, 210
Bahr, R. T., 82, 83, 90, 91
Baird, S., 135, 138
Baird Body Image Assessment Tool,
  135
Baker, J. M., 42, 46
Baker, P. O., 42, 46
Baker, W., 31, 47
Baldwin, K. A., 125, 138
Bargagliotti, L. A., 52, 67
Barnard, K., 75, 80, 90
Batzel, L., 6, 23
Baumgartner, R., 10, 23

213

Contents of Previous Volumes

VOLUME IV

ORDER FORM

Save 10% on Volume 8 with this coupon.

_____ Check here to order the ANNUAL REVIEW OF NURSING RESEARCH, Volume 8, 1990 at a 10% discount. You will recieve an invoice requesting pre-payment.

Save 10% on all future volumes with a continuation order

_____ Check here to place your continuation order for the ANNUAL REVIEW OF NURSING RESEARCH. You will recieve a pre-payment invoice with a 10% discount upon publication of each new volume, beginning with Volume 8, 1990. You may pay for prompt shipment or cancel with no obligation.

Name _____

Institution _____

Address _____

City/State/Zip _____

Examination copies for possible course adoption are available to instructors "on approval" only. Write on institutional letterhead, noting course, level, present text, and expected enrollment (Include $2.50 for postage and handling). Prices slightly higher overseas. Prices subject to change.

Mail this coupon to:
SPRINGER PUBLISHING COMPANY
536 Broadway, New York, N.Y. 10012